Integrity and Personhood

Looking at Patients from a Bio/Psycho/Social Perspective

Integrity and Personhood

Looking at Patients from a Bio/Psycho/Social Perspective

Roberta Springer Loewy
University of California, Davis
Sacramento, California

Springer Science+Business Media, LLC

ISBN 978-94-017-3846-0 ISBN 978-0-306-46827-8 (eBook)
DOI 10.1007/978-0-306-46827-8

Originally published by Kluwer Academic / Plenum Publishers, New York in 2000.
Softcover reprint of the hardcover 1st edition 2000

http://www.wkap.nl/

10 9 8 7 6 5 4 3 2 1

A C.I.P. record for this book is available from the Library of Congress

To Erich H. Loewy, my husband and professional colleague. Without Erich's wisdom, patience and unwavering faith in my potential—both as a person and as a professional—this manuscript could never have been started, much less finished. He is my empirical proof for the existence of undeserved good luck!

Preface

Since my first exposure to clinical practice in 1963 medicine has undergone quite an evolution. Back then, as I remember it, physicians were their patients' primary medical decisionmakers. That is, patients went to physicians, recited complaints, submitted to examinations and were told what particular medical intervention, according to a physician's best estimate, was required. While patients were certainly free to accept, reject or ignore their physicians' advice, their actual participation during the process of decision-making that led up to the particular medical intervention ultimately chosen was usually quite small. Obviously, the more circumspect practitioner tried to remain sensitive to the special interests and desires of each patient. But, by and large, biomedical need (as determined by the physician) was the unquestioned criterion that guided medical decisions. Back then it was simply presumed that the biomedical goals of medicine—as well as its practitioners—were obvious, unchanging and universal goods which, as a matter of course, complemented (or, at least, didn't unduly conflict with) the goals of patients. Moreover, the most efficient and fruitful means by which those goals might be reached was through the beneficent paternalism of the expert, i.e., the physician. Because opaque and remote to laypersons, such expertise was truly awe-inspiring and, even when relatively ineffective, stood largely unchallenged. As a result, the default expectation was simply that patients (and their significant others) accede to the beneficent and authoritarian expertise of their physicians.

Along with progress in science and biomedical technology, however, came the realization that, like any other cultural institution or practice, the goals of medicine are multifocal and complex. They encompass not only those vague, overarching and impersonal traditional goals of medical practice—as exemplified by our continued respect for the ancient Hippocratic admonition, "*primum non nocere*"—above all, do no harm. But they include those of a now much more culturally diverse group of medical, nursing and allied health care professionals (including all kinds of practitioners—researchers and teachers as well as clinicians) and those of an increasingly more sophisticated (and, if not more active, at least more vocal) patient population. Empirical evidence—as reflected in the public's growing dissatisfaction and distrust of medicine as a cultural institution—has made it amply clear that these goals are hardly the obvious, unchanging or universal goods they were once naively presumed to be. One need only be reminded of the Nazi and Tuskegee experiences of the recent past (and, in both cases, the unwillingness of the respective peer groups to voice objection to their colleagues' questionable activities) or, for that matter, those of the present. The continued and widespread failure of clinicians, for example, to take seriously the amount of unnecessary pain and suffering still routinely inflicted on patients today is profound. Parenthetically, throughout this work the term "clinician" will be used to refer to *any* health care professional engaged in clinical practice: physician, nurse, allied health care professional and, yes, even health care ethicist.

Of course, times *have* changed and, like the passage of time, change is inevitable. In order to survive, all living things must respond to change. In animals, this response need not be based merely on a blind impulse to react, but can be thoughtful and forward-looking as well. A hallmark feature of humans—and, I would argue, one shared in varying degrees by many other species—is the drive (for want of a better word) to guide change rather than to be guided by it. To the degree that a species is capable of consciously directing change—and doing so with foresight, prudence and understanding—it is said to be intelligent. If true, then humans ought, both singly and collectively, to be able—given the opportunity to do so—to respond with prudent and thoughtful foresight to change. The role we play—again, singly and collectively—in helping to craft a response to the changes facing medicine today ought to reflect not only our intelligence as human beings but our commitment as compassionate and caring health care clinicians as well.

While touching on the very foundations of ethics and social philosophy (and, for that reason, the interests of academics of various stripes both in and outside of the health care field) this work is, notwithstanding, written predominantly with health care clinicians in mind. That is, it is directed towards those of us still enmeshed in the daily struggle of attempting to practice our particular expertise with fidelity, compassion and intelligent foresight in the face of great and rapid changes within both our society in general and that cultural institution called "medicine" in particular. Why? Because I am convinced that we have no hope of resolving the very real and perplexing issues that confront medicine (both as a cultural institution and as a special kind of personal clinical relationship between identified individuals) today until we—individually, collectively and publicly—begin to question some very basic and widely held presuppositions in our society. Presuppositions such as these penetrate deep into the fabric of daily existence. Even being able to identify something as "a problematic situation" or "a potential resolution" is intimately connected with how persons and relationships in general are characterized. These characterizations spring from very deeply ingrained patterns of thought. They are often made "automatically," tacitly, without the benefit of critical reflection. As a result, it is imperative that the presuppositions that lie behind those characterizations be brought to light and subjected to intensely critical and ongoing public scrutiny.

Thus, a considerable portion of this book is dedicated to identifying and examining the implications of a set of common but uncritically held presuppositions about what it means to be a person. I investigate what these presuppositions are, how they come to be so readily and uncritically held and reinforced, and why their implications can have such a profound effect on how we think and act. I then argue that such presuppositions, because they are acquired without sufficient critical reflection, effectively prevent us from recognizing some crucial conditions and consequences of our unavoidable experiential existence as persons. Namely, they prevent us from recognizing that we are dynamic and interdependent "works in progress" who, in order to persist and thrive as robust individuals, must maintain a homeostatic balance in and with an equally dynamic and interdependent environment. Today's increasingly popular vision of the individual is as a radically self-made, self-sufficient, self-contained, freestanding and fully functional entity *in spite of* rather than *in light of* her bio/psycho/social context and connections. In other words, the libertarian version of the classic American ideal of the "rugged individual" is more than an exaggeration; it is a mythic fabrication that is not only internally contradictory, but counterproductive as well.

My inquiry into these uncritically held presuppositions and the problems they create and perpetuate builds on the work of the American philosopher and social critic, John Dewey. It builds, most especially, on his views concerning:

1. Logic as the theory of critical, reflective inquiry (i.e., intelligence)
2. Ethics as the intelligent use of that theory to come to a better understanding of the dynamic and evolving nature of our interrelationships with each other and our environments and, thus, to appreciate how those interrelationships define—and are defined by—commitment, obligation and responsibility
3. Democratic process as an ethical, as well as social, ideal.

While I focus more narrowly on interrelationships that exist between persons in the field of health care, the inquiry itself remains broadly philosophical in both method and content. Therefore, the conclusions I draw should not only bear directly on problems in health care, but should lead to a better understanding of persons as bio/psycho/social entities with all of the diverse needs and common, rational interests that such an embodied, situated and shared existence implies.

Acknowledgments

It is a commonplace in all disciplines that every individual's contributions rest on the shoulders of many, many others. But, of course, there are always some shoulders that are broader than others, and they are deserving of special recognition. I wish to thank my dissertation committee members from Loyola University of Chicago—Hans Seigfried, Suzanne Cunningham, David C. Thomasma—and my dissertation director and advisor, David T. Ozar for their helpful and trenchant criticisms. Especial thanks go to Dave Thomasma for giving me the opportunity to learn while teaching within his Medical Humanities Program at Loyola University of Chicago Stritch School of Medicine. Dr. Thomasma has a sense of collegiality with and professional responsibility towards his students not often evident in graduate programs. Especial thanks also go to Dave Ozar for helping me to make, from my often overly dense prose, a more coherent and rigorous account of my ideas and their implications. I would also like to thank both Dr. Sy Halleck, my reviewer with Kluwer/Plenum and Perry A. Pugno, MD, MPH, Director of the Division of Medical Education for the American Academy of Family Physicians. Their insight and suggestions were of immeasurable help in transforming what was originally a rather dense theoretical dissertation into a text more accessible to practising clinicians.

However, the broadest of shoulders have been those within my own family. Of course, they have given me the usual "moral support." But what is more important—and rewarding—they have served as my colleagues to a depth I never expected. My firstborn, Thomas R. Loewy, used his journalistic expertise to help me learn to "get to the heart of the issue," to state it as clearly as possible and to work on eliminating many of those ghastly, long-winded sentences of which philosophers are so inordinately fond. My youngest son, David M. Loewy, used his expertise in computer technology to help me understand that computers are *not* really the malignant demons I envisioned them to be.

But, by far, the finest professional colleague of my life, my severest critic, my first and still the greatest professional mentor I've ever had the privilege to observe in action is Erich Hans Loewy, now Professor and Endowed Chair of Bioethics at University of California, Davis. The genuine collegiality and loyalty Erich extends to his students and his deep and wholehearted enthusiasm for collaborative inquiry into social justice issues is truly remarkable. These traits exemplify John Dewey's notion of what ethics is really all about: a deep and abiding commitment to and responsibility for one's relationships with the rest of one's environment. These are examples of excellence of character that I will spend the remainder of a lifetime trying to emulate. It is also my incredible good fortune that Erich is not only a mentor and professional colleague, but also my partner in life.

While there were many others, without whose expertise this manuscript would never have seen the light of day, here too, there are several deserving of especial recognition. While their expertise certainly was, to paraphrase Immanuel Kant, the *means* necessary to my personal *ends* (viz., my desire to publish!), they also happen to be, each in his or her own right, wonderfully talented individuals—patient, kind and professional. Fortunately for me, they all bore my impatient inexperience with a remarkable sense of good humor—and at times I am sure this was no small feat! These individuals include Virginia Todaro and Bev Bridges from University of California Davis' Information Systems at the Sacramento campus and their technical expert counterparts at Kluwer Academic/Plenum Publishing, Gregory Safford and Robert Wheeler. Most of all, I am indebted to my editor, Mariclaire Cloutier, the Senior Editor of Medical and Behavioral Sciences at Kluwer/Plenum, for her willingness to accept this manuscript from one who has heard all of the horror stories but never before undergone the experience of book publication. I appreciate, more than any words can convey, her expert guidance and faith in my ability to succeed in this endeavor.

Contents

List of Abbreviations

N.B.: The following set of abbreviations has become the standard mode for referencing the numerous published articles, addresses, book reviews and books of John Dewey and, for the sake of both consistency and convenience, will be used throughout this work:

1. EW: *The Early Works of John Dewey, 1882-1898*. 5 vols. Edited by Jo Ann Boydston. Carbondale: Southern Illinois University Press, 1967-1972.
2. MW: *The Middle Works of John Dewey, 1899-1924*. 15 vols. Edited by Jo Ann Boydston. Carbondale: Southern Illinois University Press, 1976-1983.
3. LW: *The Later Works of John Dewey, 1925-1953*. 17 vols. Edited by Jo Ann Boydston. Carbondale: Southern Illinois University Press, 1981-1991.

Chapter 1

Introduction

1. PONDERING THE NATURE OF OBLIGATION AND RESPONSIBILITY

How we, as a community of inquirers, understand the nature of commitment, obligation and responsibility between persons is a complex phenomenon. It is determined not only by the particular surface features of any given relationship per se, but also by a number of tacit, relatively unexamined presuppositions (concerning, among other things, persons, relationships, commitments, obligations and responsibilities) that we bring to the inquiry. In turn, both of these determinations are heavily influenced by the particular social context in which we find ourselves, a context that includes interests, values and assumptions that we at least recognize, if not entirely share. And, as a social institution, how the health care professions perceive themselves depends upon much the same thing: the contexts and surface features of their relationships, the particular social context in which they find themselves and their own particular tacit, relatively unexamined presuppositions concerning persons, relationships, commitments, obligations and responsibilities.

This work is an examination of our understanding of what constitutes commitment, obligation and responsibility between patients and providers in the field of health care. It will examine this topic by looking at relevant sets of presuppositions and relevant contexts. That is, it will begin by investigating standard notions of autonomy, beneficence, non-maleficence and justice as these have been conceived in recent health care ethics literature, and by examining the actual contexts of relationships in this social institution as these materially affect and are, in turn, affected by these conceptions.

2. THE "PROFESSIONAL ETHICIST" AND THE HEALTH CARE PROFESSION

As a field that is schooled in disciplined discourse, ethics has been instrumental in recent years in helping health care professionals to grapple anew—and, I believe, to much greater effect—with ethically problematic cases. It has done this by introducing ethical theory and the philosophical tools of logic, critical thinking and conceptual analysis into the field of health care. One of the main arguments for inviting professionally trained philosophers and ethicists to reflect and comment upon the relationships between patient and health care provider is the ability of the former to provide a much needed (because quite different) additional perspective for understanding the unique contexts in which these relationships occur.

The benefit of this additional perspective derives, in part, from the fact that every person is a potential reservoir of differing and, oftentimes, novel insights about a problem. But it also derives from the fact that the kind of critical reflection practiced by ethicists and philosophers differs in both scope and intensity from the kind of critical reflection ordinarily engaged in by patients and health care providers. Among other things, ethicists working in the field of health care have been instrumental in helping everyone involved begin to see more clearly the complicated context of each health care situation, from its physical environment to its biological, emotional, aesthetic, religious, political, economic and cultural aspects. In so doing, they have helped to elucidate the multiple interconnections between these various aspects, all of which must be carefully weighed and their relevance imaginatively examined for any ethical assessment of a case to be considered thorough.

Though often reduced to the merely biological, the medical facts of any given case will—in varying degrees—affect and be affected by any or all of the above-mentioned aspects. Hence, in a full articulation of any case, every one of these aspects must be taken into consideration and carefully examined as to its relevance. Upon surviving such scrutiny, it must be included as a relevant piece of data to be incorporated into any further considerations. Of course, from the standpoint of the ethicist, the biological aspects of a case are treated as "givens" within which the remaining aspects can be examined. And correctly so: an ethicist's role with regard to the biological facts of the case is, necessarily, limited to assuring that every reasonable effort has been made to determine them correctly (e.g., that the proper specialists have been consulted and that there is enough objective data to warrant consensus among the health care professionals about diagnosis and prognosis). Only then can ethical analysis properly be said to begin.

However, from the standpoint of the health care professional, what these biological facts actually represent is merely a distillation of the field's best efforts to date in understanding very complicated physiological processes. That is, they are not simple "givens," but in reality are open to what, at times, can amount to rather wholesale modifications. In and of itself, this has never been an especially problematic matter for health care professionals themselves. Of necessity, they must quickly grow used to dealing with diagnoses, prognoses and therapies that must be established and instituted in the face of various degrees of ambiguity and uncertainty. I mention this as an important reminder that "facts" of any kind, though relatively stable for some purposes, are not permanent fixtures or universal features of existence nor need they be. Effective inquiry, like effective science, requires neither universality nor absolute certainty but can—and, in fact, must—rely on the judicious use of statistical probability in the face of idiosyncratic findings.

So, in regard to the biological facts of the case, the role of the ethicist—much like that of the patient—is necessarily relatively passive. This is so, not because biological facts about any given patient are utterly fixed or universal laws of nature. Rather, it is because some participants to the conversation (in this case health care providers) are more qualified to establish the relative relevance of certain kinds of facts to the case by virtue of their exposure to and deliberate cultivation of an intensely focused set of experiences and interpretations. Thus, the ethicist—just like the patient—must place her trust in and rely upon the expertise of clinicians for a realistic assessment of the biological "facts" of the case. (Analogously, what the ethicist hopes for is a similar flexibility and openness to new understanding regarding the ethical and other contextual features of health care situations, new understanding that will grow as the ethicist's special skills are honed and refined through practice.)

One place where these biological aspects of a case can become ethically problematic is in health care providers' communication (and lack of communication) of them, of their consequences, and of the implications of their consequences to patients and their stipulated significant others. They can become problematic because the biological facts of a case belong to a person, i.e., a rational, sentient entity that necessarily exists within—and thus cannot possibly be understood in complete isolation from—an environment. That is, biological facts "belong to" a person in the sense that, though they are physiological data, their precise meanings depend upon how the patient understands and incorporates that data. That is, it depends upon how this data will affect her daily life and her understanding of herself as the primary author, as it were, of that life. Hence, a realistic assessment of and meaning for these biological facts in this particular situation cannot develop without the existence of an engaged, on-going dialogue between health care providers and patient (or designated other).

Certainly, ethicists have made a major contribution in this particularly problematic area by helping health care providers become more aware of their obligation to communicate these biological facts, and to do so as sensitively, confidentially and unambiguously as possible. By means of this contribution, patients have a greater opportunity for making intelligent, well-informed decisions about their own health care and for maximizing their participation in that care.

As for the psychological (including emotional and religious) aspects of a case, here too, ethicists have made important contributions to the thinking of health care providers and their patients. That is, they have assisted both patients and their care-givers to develop more imagination, sensitivity and responsiveness in identifying and understanding personal interests, values and needs—their own as well as those of others. This has encouraged a more active, responsible and balanced collaboration between health care providers and patients. Ethicists have also assisted health care providers in developing more effective conceptual tools for critically analysing and discussing such things as, for example, what constitutes decisional capacity in each particular patient or what presumed consent and informed consent are, how they differ and why.

Unfortunately, a third set of aspects are often more difficult to examine—for ethicists and for health care providers and patients alike. These are the social aspects that include political, religious, economic and any other cultural aspects of human existence. While ethicists have sometimes contributed to articulating social aspects in problematic cases, this move is not common because of the sets of concepts—and the presuppositions on which they rest—that most contemporary health care ethicists employ. Even when made, it has usually been by abandoning the analysis of particular, concrete cases and by moving in a different direction. That is, the move has been to sort cases in terms of whether they are issues of micro- or macro-allocation, and then to treat these issues as though they exist entirely unconnected to and unaffected by one another.

Without doubt, this approach has led to some extremely helpful distinctions for certain kinds of analyses—especially in areas that concern political and economic institutions. All too often, however, it has led to treating large scale social structures (e.g., the various professions, health care institutions, economic institutions and various public associations and affiliations generally) as though the problems they confront could be addressed in isolation from day-to-day health care encounters instead of seeing these encounters as particular, concrete problems that occur within and are unavoidably connected to and shaped by the larger social and cultural frameworks.

This particular way of dealing with social issues in health care has often had another unfortunate effect. Namely, it has led many ethicists, as well as the patients and health care providers they serve, to treat the social aspects of particular cases as though they were analogues of biological "givens" in a case. That is, they are treated as features to be passively accepted rather than regarded as changeable, ethically significant and deserving of careful attention at the same time the more local details of the cases are being considered. For both ethicists and health care providers alike (and I include psychiatrists and psychologists here as well), the social aspects of a case are too often treated as unalterable conditions beyond discussion at the bedside (i.e., at the micro-level) instead of material circumstances that are the product of prior *social* (i.e., macro-level) negotiation—even if they now are treated with tacit acquiescence—and, for that reason alone, still eminently negotiable. Since there is, as yet, little that can be modified concerning the circumstances of our biology in comparison to what can, potentially, be modified concerning the social circumstances of our lives, the biological and the social aspects are clearly not analogous in this respect and should not be treated as such.

This persistent disanalogy is the reason for the dissatisfaction felt towards a particular class of health care ethics cases by ethicists and health care providers alike; namely, cases in which they are struggling to articulate and to examine those alternatives available to patients and their families or significant others. These alternatives are those that are located at the interface between the needs of individual patients and the values and priorities of the community, as these are represented by specific institutions within the community.[1]

3. THE FOCUS OF THIS WORK

This text will focus on an examination of cases of this sort, in which elements of social context play a pivotal role in the ethical issues at stake but which are, nonetheless, often overlooked or assumed to be unchangeable "givens," with little or no argument. In other words, I will argue that the standard ways in which health care ethicists, health care providers and patients have tended to discuss and to analyse ethical issues in health care have not adequately addressed the possibility that social elements of a situation are *not* beyond examination, critical analysis and collaborative reconstruction. Ethicists and health care providers alike have been inappropriately passive before these social aspects. This is why there can be little doubt that this area of concern would profit from even greater input from ethics as a discipline.

My focus in this work will be to construct, test and defend an alternative to the approaches typically taken in the ethical analyses of such cases. Thus, I will provide some cases that are representative of this problem and, examining these cases carefully, I will first show how the approaches that I am criticizing address them, and then explain not only what these approaches miss but, more importantly, why they miss it. I will then demonstrate that these approaches typically involve presuppositions about persons, relationships, obligations and responsibilities that leave them unable to take adequate account of the social/contextual features of a case. Their inability to inform us adequately about such cases, I will argue, is grounded in these defective presuppositions. In defending this view, I will, in other words, be challenging some rather basic assumptions commonly made in contemporary health care ethics concerning persons and the nature of their relatedness.

For the sake of having a convenient name for the forms of ethical analysis that I will be criticizing here, I will refer to them collectively as "the standard approach." The sets of concepts and modes of ethical analysis that I intend by this phrase will be illustrated in detail in chapter two. There I will show how "the standard approach" deals with problematic cases in such as way as to highlight this approach's defects. In calling this "the standard approach" I am not, of course, claiming that all contemporary health care ethicists practice it or that ethicists who employ other such concepts, presuppositions and modes of inquiry to issues in health care are automatically therefore considered inept. But by a significant margin, the approach that I am calling "the standard approach" is the most common way in which issues are currently discussed in the health care ethics literature and have been discussed for nearly two decades.

Hence, the appellation, "standard approach," is well deserved. That it *is* so typical, however, is not the concern of this work, which is written from a perspective that is philosophical rather than merely sociological. The concern to be addressed here is that this pattern of inquiry is seriously defective. It is built on presuppositions that leave it essentially blind, and therefore passive, to the impact of ethically important social/contextual features of health care situations. And this is what shall concern us here.

4. THE BROADER IMPLICATIONS OF THE PROJECT

While I will be looking specifically at problematic relationships between persons in the setting of health care, the basic assumptions that I challenge are certainly more fundamental insofar as they form the basis of how we often think about persons and the nature of human interreactions in general. My investigation will show how these assumptions affect other related background assumptions, shaping attitudes and conduct towards a set of concepts about persons that includes (though it is not necessarily limited to) autonomy, beneficence, non-maleficence and justice.

There are a number of good reasons why someone interested in sorting out various presuppositions about persons and their connectedness would benefit from analysing the relationship between providers and recipients of health care. Of course, such a move is hardly novel. The Greek philosopher, Plato (circa 300 BCE), for example, thought that one of the best ways to get clear about the "soul" is to look at the actual relationship of citizens to the polis which he treated as an inquiry into the "health" of the soul. But there are other, more important reasons for using the health care context to raise questions concerning common presuppositions about relationships, obligations and responsibilities.

First, there is a distinctive combination of intimacy and distance characteristic of relationships between providers and recipients of health care. For this reason, health care provides a richer context for studying relationships than settings wherein only one or other of these characteristics are evident. In other words, because health care relationships share aspects of both the intimacy evident in personal relationships and the detachment characteristic of impersonal relationships—at least as they are currently understood in our culture—they seem to be an exceptionally good place to focus a study of common presuppositions about relationships.

Second, there is already an ongoing discussion among philosophers interested in health care about the appropriate model(s) of relationship health care should aspire to or adopt. Working in this area will provide an important "head start," since this study will be able to add to our understanding without having to initiate the inquiry *de novo*.

Third, my own past experience as a health care provider (specifically as a registered nurse with more than fifteen years of experience ranging from geriatric to intensive care practice) can bring to such a project a familiarity with and, hopefully, a better understanding of certain aspects of the health care setting. This will help to focus the examination of these presuppositions on concrete, real life aspects of relationship and social context. An important risk of a foundational study of presuppositions and context in ethical reflection lies in its becoming too abstract and, thus, too difficult to translate back to the ordinary details of life. By focusing this philosophic inquiry on the health care setting, I hope to keep its reflections more concrete, precise and, therefore, more accessible to both professionals and non-professionals alike.

Finally, for John Dewey, whose philosophical work has guided much of my method in general, and this project in particular, the test of any theory—philosophical or otherwise—is whether it actually helps in the resolution of a pressing problem. Should the results of my inquiry help to clarify some aspects of the knotty problems in health care associated with the complicated bio/psycho/social dynamics of persons then, according to Dewey, the value of the project would be empirically demonstrated.

5. METHODOLOGY

This project utilizes an alternative methodology based on the critical and experimental attitude of reflective inquiry advocated by John Dewey.[2] That is, it is a methodology that is critical, empirical, experimental, pragmatic, naturalistic, pluralistic and non-reductionistic. While Dewey's contributions to this project will be explained more fully in chapter three, each of these terms deserves, for the moment, a brief explanation. The method of this project is *critical* in the self-corrective sense that all reflection (including philosophic reflection) is treated as a scientific investigation of "causal antecedents and causative consequents,"[3] seminal features in any inquiry. It is *empirical* and *experimental* in the sense that it begins with lived experience which it then subjects to a systematic accumulation of evidence through the deliberate modification, transformation and reconstruction of the antecedent material of that experience.[4] That is, it appeals to a scientific investigation of experience instead of attempting to posit some hypothetical account of human nature as an heuristic device

The method of this project is *pragmatic* in the sense that experience is treated as an ongoing series of dynamic interactions—what Dewey called "a matter of *simultaneous* doings and sufferings"—between each living being and its physical and social environment.[5] Consequences, when they are operationally instituted[6] with due care, will function as tests of the validity of the results of critical reflection on these interactions. Thus, reflective inquiry is treated as an inherently public, social activity, an activity that is cumulative, self-correcting and evolving, an activity that has distinctive survival value for its practitioners, both individually and collectively.

The method of this project is *naturalistic* in the following senses: (1) it holds that there is a common logical pattern of knowing in science and morals;[7] (2) it rejects the belief that experience is some mysterious thing external, but somehow attached, to a living being;[8] and (3) it treats experience as a complex, evolving field within which each living being is a dynamic, interactive component within an equally dynamic, interactive environment.[9, 10] That is, such a methodology targets, critically analyses and suggests a way of reconstructing presuppositions that ignore an unalterable aspect of the actual situatedness of persons: namely, that persons are fragile, responsive "works in progress"—simultaneously products and agents who, in order to preserve their integrity *as persons*, must maintain a dynamic homeostatic balance within an equally fragile and responsive environment.

Finally, the method of this project is *pluralistic* and, therefore, *non-reductionistic* in the sense that, because persons are bio/psycho/social entities, what characterizes them *as individual and unique persons* cannot be reduced to any one of these aspects alone—as, for example, the biological aspect of "being alive." Rather, persons are said to "have lives," which requires attention to the entire bio/psycho/social field of their existences.[11] Because the experience of persons is an unavoidably bio/psycho/social phenomenon, efforts to increase our understanding of that phenomenon should be pursued in bio/psycho/social terms. That is, what counts as inquiry, evidence and explanation cannot ignore and will be integrally tied to learning how the bio/psycho/social aspects of experiences dynamically interreact. According to this view, *all* concepts central to persons will be unavoidably and irreducibly bio/psycho/social.

So, in general, how to proceed? The project borrows, at every level of inquiry, a stratagem favored by Plato's Socrates. Plato initiated a number of his dialogues with Socrates hailing a friend or group of acquaintances by way of two questions: "Where have you come from?" and "Where are you going?"[12] These queries pointed beyond the merely geographical. They served as foils for the purpose of introducing the personalities of the interlocutors and establishing the precise context and development of a problematic issue—everything relevant from the brute, physical features to its more abstract, intellectual ones. A dialogue then ensued about the meaning of that problematic issue, wherein a variety of alternatives were solicited and offered—sometimes timidly, sometimes brashly, often enthusiastically, but always in a surprisingly democratic spirit—in answer to a third, usually unarticulated question: "How do we get there?" These three questions are basic, time-honored questions that structure virtually all intelligible and intelligent inquiry into the most abstract, theoretical, practical and/or mundane of situations or issues.[13] Such inquiry, when controlled, can transform experiences that are indeterminate into experiences that are, to paraphrase Dewey, funded with meaning.

The first question, "Where have you come from?" establishes the historical context of the inquiry—the past physical environment, biological parameters and psychosocial elements that enter into a situation or issue—in order that its presuppositions may be revealed and assessed. The second question, "Where are you going?" investigates the "destination" or future of an inquiry, its meaning, its various aims, its possible consequences and the intentions, presuppositions and commitments of those who initiate and those who stand to benefit from it. The third question, "How do we get there?" prompts the marshalling of various plans of action, the means by which tentative responses to the second question might be approximated and tested.

Each of these three questions must be asked and answered sequentially in any controlled inquiry. Moreover, a lack of answers or paucity of solutions to the third question may necessitate a renegotiation of what constitutes an acceptable answer to the second. It may even necessitate a reassessment of the first. While such to-and-fro assessments and re-evaluations serve to hone the inquiry by clarifying its meaning and the various available options and their consequences, they do not change the basic structure of this pattern of inquiry. Indeed, any intelligent inquiry, whether the subject matter is science or morals, must ask and answer these three basic questions in one way or another. By maintaining this pattern, the goals and expectations of the inquiry are kept realistic and appropriate.

The characteristics of reflective inquiry that are embodied by these three questions are, in fact, the basis for Dewey's claim that, for critical, reflective thought to succeed, it must rely on the method of science.[14] For Dewey believed that the actual method of scientific inquiry is the best example we have yet developed of intelligence at work. This method is not the same as the pseudoscience that passes for so much of what is popularly considered scientific thought—a narrow, technical view of science in which changeless laws are discovered, memorized and externally applied. Rather, the method espoused here is the same continuous, progressive, democratic and collaborative process (including its painstakingly controlled and monitored antecedents and consequents) that occurs in laboratories, field work, and wherever communities of researchers wholeheartedly and co-operatively work together, imaginatively anticipating and offering alternative resolutions to actual problems of living.

6. SUMMARY OF REMAINING CHAPTERS

In chapter two a number of select cases are presented in order to provide a careful analysis of how ethical issues in health care are standardly conceived and discussed today. In the course of this presentation, certain inadequacies in the standard approach become evident and prompt the following question: why is it that so much is overlooked in how the issues are conceived and discussed? It is proposed that these inadequacies occur because the standard approach in question relies on moral theories that are themselves based on presuppositions that are open to serious question; and it is suggested that this difficulty can be addressed with the help of John Dewey.

Chapter three is devoted to an examination of the key elements that my project shares with John Dewey's pragmatic and naturalistic methodological approach. The purpose of such an examination is to help make explicit some of my own central assumptions and to provide cogent reasons in their defense. To that end, Dewey's theory of experience is reviewed. Next, a detailed analysis of his account of reflective inquiry is undertaken in order to clarify much of the approach and some of the substantive claims developed later in this work.

In particular, Dewey understood reflective inquiry to be the method of intelligence, and described it as a complex, evolutionary and inherently collective (i.e., public and social) activity that has distinctive survival value for its individual practitioners. For Dewey the capacity to engage in such reflective inquiry is what characterizes us as beings capable of understanding the nature of our relationships with the rest of the world, including the importance of social contexts and how these affect and are affected by how we perceive ourselves as persons.

Also addressed in chapter three is Dewey's view of science as a paradigm for the method of critical inquiry. He reminds us that reflective inquiry is something that is done and not simply thought. Moreover, the melioristic character of reflective inquiry that follows from treating intelligence as a process that is both perspectival (because pursued by unique individuals) and falsifiable (because pursued freely and in open collaboration) is noted. By enhancing our ability to "have a hand" in our progress both as individuals and as participants in a community, reflective inquiry is the process by which we come to understand commitments, obligations and responsibilities and, thus, to recognize our uniqueness as ethical beings.

In chapter four, certain key presuppositions of the ethical theories on which the standard approach to health care ethics rests are challenged. These key presuppositions—especially a much-vaunted notion of autonomy as an isolated, insulated locus of rational self-determination and self-sufficiency—are central to the way personhood is standardly conceived. These key presuppositions are analysed, criticized, reconstructed and carefully qualified in Deweyian terms. As part of this process, the following material conditions of persons are examined: (1) that throughout their lives persons experience basic needs[15] which, when unmet, cause them to suffer and (2) that persons, whether they consciously appreciate their situation or not, depend on others for the prevention or amelioration of some portion of their own suffering.

These material conditions strongly suggest that a person's experience is shaped by interdependence. By virtue of the fact that it permeates the very existence—if not the conscious experience—of all persons, interdependence is thus construed to be a standard characteristic of personhood. Therefore, we are justified in viewing persons as bio/psycho/social beings from our first efforts to understand them.

Moreover, if interdependence is thus considered a significant characteristic and not simply a *defect* of persons, then it should also be considered a significant factor in determining what constitutes persons as autonomous agents. This conclusion, however, runs counter to the prevailing assumptions about personhood in the ethical theories that underpin the current health care ethics approach. The prevalent view has been to set autonomy in simple opposition to heteronomy, thus effectively minimizing or ignoring the consequences and implications of the fundamentally interdependent existence of persons. In other words, if interdependence is a central feature of personhood, then these ethical theories must have something more to say about its role in human agency, responsibility and obligation. The antecedents and consequents of interdependence—including the influence that suffering from unmet basic needs has on the development of our understanding of what ethical obligation amounts to—will be taken more seriously here. Thus a more viable starting point from which to understand these ethical relationships between persons will be made available.

In chapter five the cases analysed in chapter two by the standard approach used in health care ethics today are re-examined from the Deweyian perspective articulated in chapters three and four. This will serve to illustrate what a bio/psycho/social understanding of ethical obligation amounts to and how it operates. An analysis of these case analyses is then, in turn, undertaken in order to identify, test and then assess the methodological approach proposed, employed and defended herein.

In the concluding section of chapter five, the bio/psycho/social interpretation of personhood developed in this work is compared to the static, self-contained and oppositional rendering of personhood that characterizes the standard approach. This comparison reveals that, because it is more sensitive to the delicate, yet dynamic, homeostatic mechanisms that preserve the integrity of persons in their relationships with their environment, a bio/psycho/social approach offers a more flexible means for resolving specific problematic situations. It should, therefore, be adopted as the most productive approach presently available to us for health care ethics;

that is, for applying the full powers of human intelligence to the ethical issues that arise in health care.

ENDNOTES

1. John Dewey would identify this dissatisfaction as the first step, however inchoate, in the progression common to all inquiry: the perception of an indeterminate "hitch" in the flow of experience. This hitch becomes more determinate—i.e., it takes on more clarity and definition—during the process of inquiry. See *LW* 12:108-11 in the chapter entitled, "The Pattern of Inquiry."
2. For Dewey's most comprehensive treatment of reflective inquiry, see his 1938 work, *Logic: The Theory of Inquiry*, *LW* 12. Alternatively, one can get a sense of what Dewey was up to from a careful reading of his article, "Logical Conditions of a Scientific Treatment of Morality." This article, though written in 1903, was included with only minor revisions in a 1946 collection of essays entitled, *Problems of Men,* (New York: Philosophical Library, 1946, pp. 211-49.) See *MW* 3:3-39.
3. For Dewey, the moment we begin thinking about and discussing immediate experience, it is the means-consequence relationship that is being considered. That is, we evaluate immediate experience in terms of its relationships—the conditions that mediate it and the things that it, in turn, mediates. *LW* 1:297; 301-2.
4. *LW* 14:14-25.
5. *MW* 10:6-9.
6. *LW* 12:4.
7. *LW* 14:62. Like Dewey, I wish to avoid what he criticized as "knowing in the orthodox sense," by which he meant an accommodation of self and its beliefs to conditions already fixed.
8. *LW* 14:17.
9. *LW* 16:108-9.
10. A brief explanation is in order here concerning my use of the term, "interactive." Dewey ascribed very precise functions to the terms, "self-action," "inter-action" and "trans-action." According to his notion of self-action, "things are viewed as acting under their own powers." Inter-action is the term Dewey used to describe a relationship "where thing is balanced against thing in causal interconnection." My use of interaction is actually closest to Dewey's use of trans-action: "where systems of description and naming [as opposed to 'things' or 'entities'] are employed to deal with aspects and phases of action, without final attribution to 'elements' or other presumptively detachable or independent 'entities,' 'essences,' or 'realities,' and without isolation of presumptively detachable 'relations' from such detachable 'elements.' " (*LW* 16:101-4) I choose to avoid the term, "transaction," itself however, because of its prominent association today with exchange relationships in the marketplace. This current association fails to capture the transformative, evolutionary characteristics of the relationships that Dewey intended to convey by using the term, "transaction." In order to avoid this unintended association, I use either of two terms—"interaction" and "interreaction"—to convey Dewey's sense of the term, "transaction."
11. The distinction I draw between "being alive" and "having a life" will be explained in the section entitled *Zoe and Bios* in chapter four.
12. The most explicit example is the first lines uttered by Socrates in the "Phaedrus," but these three questions are asked or answered by Socrates in other dialogues including

"Euthyphro," "Ion," "Theaetetus," and more obliquely in the "Protagoras" and "Timaeus."

13. This strategy has been adapted, refined, used and taught as a method of ethics consultation and medical case presentation for at least ten years now by Erich Loewy in his health care ethics programs. With his permission I have drawn liberally from his experiences and expertise in my description of this methodology.
14. *MW* 6:69ff, 177ff; *MW* 12:172ff.
15. Much has been written in ethics literature concerning what constitutes a basic need. It is beyond the scope of this work to argue for a particular view. For the purposes of the work, I will simply assume basic needs to be those needs necessary (1) to maintain biological existence (what I describe in chapter four as "zoe," or "being alive") and (2) to provide an equal opportunity to access those materials/resources that make it possible to pursue and develop a biographical existence (what I describe in chapter four as "bios," or "having a life.")

Chapter 2

Case Presentations and Standard Analyses

1. INTRODUCTION

The following cases will be examined via a format of analysis that is considered standard in both the literature and practice of health care ethics today. It follows the format described in chapter one: the biological and pathophysiological aspects of the case will be examined, followed by the psychological, and then the social aspects of the case. While investigating these aspects and how the various participants in the case understand and value their implications, the central conflicting issues of the case and the benefits and drawbacks of the alternative courses of action for resolving them will be identified and discussed.

In a standard case analysis, a course of action is then chosen to resolve these conflicts. The ideals, goals, characteristics and values that this course of action is thought to preserve or promote are expressed in principles that, in turn, are offered to explain and/or to justify the preferred decision or course of action. Among the main principles standardly invoked in health care ethics today are autonomy, beneficence, non-maleficence and justice. The best known source for this standard approach and the four principles it utilizes is Beauchamp's and Childress' *Principles of Biomedical Ethics*.[1] It is the approach that has dominated the Georgetown summer workshops that have introduced so many participants to discussion of issues in health care ethics.

The approach to health care ethics that these four principles are here used to typify has many other sources and representations in the contemporary practice of health care ethics. Though widely advocated, this approach has a number of critics; however, few of them challenge the presuppositions of the approach in the manner to be proposed here. Still, the widespread currency of this approach is common knowledge within the field of health care ethics, which is why its presuppositions are deserving of the careful examination offered here.

Using this standard approach, three cases will be analysed in this chapter with a view towards examining the merits, and especially the demerits, of this approach. In chapter five, these cases will be re-examined in order to explain how the corrected presuppositions about persons and their bio/psycho/social interdependence that are developed in the intervening chapters significantly alter our understanding of both (a) the nature and scope of the obligations between patients and health care professionals in the three cases and (b) the principles and goals of health care practice that inform these obligations.

Before turning to the case analyses, these four principles, as they are standardly conceived, need a brief introduction. Obviously, because volumes have been—and will continue to be—written about each of these principles and the often times conflicting values they embody, this brief introduction makes no pretensions of giving a comprehensive picture of any one of these notions. Such a picture would, in any event, be quite beyond the scope and focus of my particular interest here. That these principles continue to be so widely discussed and debated can only lend support to my contention that the way they are currently conceived and used can actually hamper, rather than enhance, the controlled inquiry needed for there to be well-crafted resolutions to problematic situations.

2. PRINCIPLES STANDARDLY INVOKED IN HEALTH CARE ETHICS

2.1 Beneficence and Non-maleficence

The Hippocratic oath, a pledge still taken by many upon entrance into the field of medicine, is symbolic of the important role that the ethical principles of beneficence and non-maleficence play in contemporary western culture. These principles have been given extensive treatment in classic texts dealing with the philosophical bases of health care ethics.[2-5] A famous injunction derived from that oath—strive to help, but above all, do no harm—influences the professional practice of all health care professionals today. It does so precisely because it confronts the ambiguous character of expertise and its consequences: the greater the power to help, the greater the possibility to do harm.

The last half of that injunction—above all, do no harm—is the basis of the principle of non-maleficence. The injunction serves as a reminder that actions always have consequences and that agents are largely responsible for the consequences of their actions *even when those consequences extend beyond the agents' intentions or expectations*. The first part of that injunction—strive to help—forms the basis of the principle of beneficence. By means of their special expertise, health care professionals strive to help their patients. Of course, this "help" can take many forms, from disinterested offering of advice to actual appropriation of decision-making responsibilities for a patient. A significant part of the ongoing dialogue about beneficence in the health care literature is an attempt to determine how to distinguish clearly between actions that are beneficent and those that are not by addressing the issue of what constitutes helping patients—and by whose definition.

2.2 Justice

While the principle of justice has been conceived from a number of conflicting perspectives,[6] these various conceptions do have certain features in common: (a) that justice is obligatory and not simply optional and (b) that justice is concerned with giving persons what is their due. Of course, what is in dispute between these conflicting conceptions of justice is how to determine what constitutes "obligation" *vis à vis* what constitutes "due." However, any discussion of "obligation" or "due," in turn, rides piggy-back on a determination of what constitutes "persons" and what it is that makes them autonomous which, because it is also a matter of dispute, hardly provides more clarity to the issue.

In a great majority of health care ethics cases analysed today, the way in which the notion of justice is customarily perceived—as my sample cases are intended to show—begins by isolating the individual or individuals involved. That is, it emphasizes a view of persons as self-sufficient and self-contained. This, in turn, significantly affects the way in which the scope of the notions of obligation and due is interpreted.

2.3 Autonomy

The last—but hardly least—principle to be examined is that of autonomy, which requires that persons be respected and which is intimately connected to the notions of liberty and self-determination. The principle of autonomy finds its classic expression in the version of Immanuel Kant's categorical imperative wherein persons are required to treat each other never merely as means, but always at the same time as ends in themselves.[7] Because it underwrites an important, albeit imprecise, set of characteristics thought to be central to persons, the principle of autonomy has been invoked both to defend and to condemn all sorts of interactions between persons. Take, for example, the issue of paternalism—i.e., treating patients without their informed and willing consent and justifying such treatment on the basis of a professional obligation to benefit one's patients—which continues to loom so large as an issue in health care practice. The principle of autonomy has been invoked both in criticism against and in defense of paternalism.

On the one side, it has acted as a counterbalance to a belief still shared by many health care professionals: namely, the belief that their special expertise makes them more qualified to determine what is in the best interests of patients than patients themselves. Opponents of this belief use the principle of autonomy to argue that persons must be presumed to be capable of making their own decisions. Some of them even argue that the only obligation experts have is to make available their expertise, which persons might then freely choose to ignore, heed or disregard. On the other side, the principle of autonomy has been appropriated to mount one of the strongest defenses for paternalism: a justification of paternalistic actions based on the claim that such actions constitute the only means available for preserving or re-establishing a patient's autonomy. Invoking the principle of autonomy, these thinkers argue that special expertise not merely permits but, under certain conditions, *obligates* experts to engage in paternalistic practices.

As can be seen by this brief introductory discussion, the same principle can be, and often is, invoked in support of opposing sides of an issue. This suggests that it is not these ethical principles themselves that are so central to the decision-making process. Instead, it suggests that there is something else behind these ethical principles (viz., ethical intuitions) which, when left unexamined, will influence the direction and outcome of that process in ways that cannot be anticipated. Certainly, without unexamined ethical intuitions of some sort, the decision-making process could never get off the ground. But, unless our unexamined ethical intuitions undergo the same careful scrutiny to which the rest of the process is subjected, there is no way to understand or to assess the role they play or, more importantly, their influence over us. The case analyses presented in this chapter illustrate how an over-reliance on ethical principles can actually hinder discovery of and reflective inquiry into the role that these important ethical intuitions play in decision-making.

3. A BRIEF LOOK AT THE ROLE ETHICAL PRINCIPLES PLAY IN CASE RESOLUTION

In order to clarify how ethical principles are used and what aspect of them is emphasized in standard case analyses, a representative description of such principles will be examined. Glen C. Graber and David C. Thomasma provide the one offered here in Theory and Practice in Medical Ethics:

> Moral principles express fundamental theoretical norms...A moral principle is an ought-statement which may express (or yield) a command about (imperative), a precept towards (prescriptive), or a description of (descriptive) conduct to be done or avoided.[8]

This definition implies, among other things, the idea that principles, like rules, are "summary," insofar as they are useful in summarizing antecedent cultural behaviors and practices and their outcomes. That is to say, they are useful, shorthand formulations that convey how problems presently faced have been addressed successfully in the past. Such a summary description of principles easily lends itself to support a kind of formalistic interpretation of principles, values, rules or theories consistent with an *applications* model of problem-solving, i.e., a predominantly top-down strategy that applies concepts to specific issues or particular cases. This formalistic interpretation is presupposed in much problem-solving that occurs in the field of health care ethics today, irrespective of whether the actual theory behind the activity of problem-solving is predominantly deductivist, dialectical, principlist, casuistical or situationalist.[9]

One of the weaknesses of the applications model is that it can too easily lull the problem-solver into thinking of the disposition of a case as "solved" rather than "resolved," two words that can be used to capture an important distinction. That is, "solving" a case by the application of principles is suggestive of a discrete and circumscribed activity comparable to, and often defined in terms of, an externally imposed intervention that has a fairly clearly demarcated beginning and end. Moreover, the intervening agent remains insulated from and unaffected by whatever actions are required by the "solution." Such a portrayal of problem solving can encourage closure of such finality or definitiveness that the further consequences that inevitably flow from a case and its disposition are all but ignored.

However, to "resolve" a case carries with it connotations of progressive, *mutual* re-adjustment. That is, it is a re-adjustment in the sense that it affects and is affected by *every* aspect of the case—including all of those persons—be they agents or patients—who are involved. It is a "resolution" insofar as it suggests a developmental reworking through a problematic situation. Such a reworking requires careful attendance to the problematic situation's discrete context and its possible solutions. It also requires maintaining an openness to the inevitable and ongoing ramifications of the solutions' consequences in light of these mutual re-adjustments and the internal dynamics of the situation itself. Such problem solving by *resolution* describes Dewey's evolutionary activity of making an indeterminate situation more determinate.[10]

In contrast to the top-down strategy of the applications approach that will be used to solve the cases in this chapter, *resolution* (as it has been outlined here and will be utilized in the reconstructed cases in chapter five) is more stringent. It requires, at minimum, openness to the reciprocal interreaction between principles as tentative guides (*not* as stipulations) and the rest of the progressive and experiential context of a problematic case. That is, it denies that a solution can be found *via* a systematic execution of a predetermined principle or algorithm. Instead, what is required is *resolution*, which necessitates (a) openness to the experiential context of a problematic situation, (b) attention to the variety of possibilities that principles can represent and (c) acknowledgement of the progressive effect that the particular development of a case has on future practice and behavior, both individual and institutional.

A standard objection against an applications model runs as follows: since no rule, principle or theory has ever been shown to be adequate or complete, there is no independent mechanism to be "applied," and thus, no solutions to practical issues can be deduced. The objection offered in this work is more fundamental: it denies the possibility of an independent mechanism that can be "applied" by denying the presumption that either "things" (be they material or conceptual) or their meanings can have freestanding or isolated existences. Since no "thing" exists in a vacuum, neither can its meaningfulness. That is, things that exist (whether that existence is material or conceptual), exist only within a bio/psycho/social context. This bio/psycho/social context provides the setting within which an implicit meaning of a thing is represented by the way it functions within that context.[11] As such, things are necessarily interconnected bio/psycho/social phenomena.

Prime examples of complex material and/or conceptual "things," are means and ends-in-view: they are always context-dependent. Because they are generated in discrete situations by individuals who are particular and distinctive members of a shared bio-social context, what is treated as an end-in-view in one situation (or even in different aspects of the same situation) functions as a means to some other end-in-view in another situation (or different aspect of the same situation). In short: their meanings depend on context. Therefore, descriptions such as Thomasma's and Graber's do not address merely the summary aspect of principles, but their practical aspect as well. Once this practical aspect of principles is taken into account, the top-down strategy of the "applications" model is eclipsed by the requirement that principles, like rules and theories, must continually be tested for their adequacy by their actual or hypothetically anticipated practical implications (i.e., by their future consequents) and not the other way around (i.e., by their antecedent conditions alone—which, of course, includes consequences, but these are the consequences of past experience). However, gaining an understanding of how these two approaches and their implications differ is best accomplished in the course of actual case analysis, and it is to this activity that we must now turn.

4. CASE ANALYSES

4.1 The "Rescue Medicine" Conundrum

During a recent cold winter an indigent, elderly man was brought into a local emergency room with pneumonia. He was close to starvation and suffered from hypothermia because he could not afford to eat or heat his room after paying his rent. While in the emergency room, the man suffered a cardiac arrest and was stabilized after aggressive cardio-pulmonary resuscitation. But, after three weeks, he remained completely unresponsive and totally dependent on a ventilator. During this time social services discovered that the man had no family or friends. The health care team suspected that the patient would remain permanently comatose, and a neurological consult confirmed the team's suspicion that the patient's prognosis was bleak.

An ethicist was consulted to discuss whether it was ethically appropriate to discontinue this man's treatment and was told by the health care team that between $100,000 and $200,000 had been expended treating this man. The health care team members concurred that, had it been possible to restore the patient to a semblance of his pre-hospitalization condition (which it was not), they would have felt no qualms about continuing treatment. Such treatment would have, in effect, returned this patient to the material conditions responsible for his hospitalization in the first place.[11]

4.1.1 Analysis

The biological facts of this case are fairly straightforward, and had the neurological status of the patient been unclear, prognosis could have been further corroborated by blood flow studies of the brain. These studies can, because of their high degree of accuracy, help to classify patients into three rather clearly defined categories: brain-dead, permanently comatose and persistently vegetative. A patient is classified as brain-dead when no blood flow to the brain can be visualized. (In all fifty states, brain death is considered the legal equivalent of the death of the person. This makes it legally acceptable to withdraw life support without fear of being charged with patient abandonment or homicide.)

A patient becomes a candidate for inclusion under the second category when there is blood flow to the brain but, after being stabilized, the patient remains completely unresponsive even to deep, painful stimuli. The person to whom this has occurred is most likely, after three weeks, permanently comatose. Patients falling into the third category exhibit what appear to be episodes of waking and sleeping but otherwise remain unresponsive. In this condition, there is blood flow to the brain but either it is insufficient or it has, at some point, been interrupted long enough to cause severe damage to or destruction of those areas of the brain associated with the "higher," or cognitive functions so characteristic of persons. Patients such as these, after being stabilized, will remain in what is called a persistent or permanently vegetative state. So long as individuals can be stabilized on life support—i.e., so long as oxygenated blood can be circulated to the cells of the body—their vegetative functions (i.e., those involuntary functions of glands and organs that are controlled by the sympathetic and parasympathetic nervous systems) can be artificially assisted indefinitely.

There are psychological facts about this case that are troubling. It is known only that this patient is—and will remain—unable to speak for himself, that he has no family or friends and that he has been living in extreme poverty. Social services have researched his case for any further data that might be helpful, but have been unable to learn any information that might prove helpful in piecing together the man's history. Thus there is no concrete idea of what his wishes might have been concerning continuation or withdrawal of life-extending treatment under these circumstances. In effect, this patient's previous isolation and poverty, along with his present condition of health and current inability to communicate, to judge or to make choices have made it a practical impossibility to anticipate how he would have chosen for himself regarding this situation.

The social aspects of this case are, by standard analysis, fairly straightforward. Because health care is such an important culturally shared value, clinicians are committed by their respective professional codes of ethics to treat each patient under their care with respect. This commitment to patients has long been reflected in formal statements about the primary goals and values of health care professionals, which have traditionally included:

1. Curing whenever possible
2. Relieving pain and alleviating symptoms
3. Maintaining/improving function and minimizing loss of function
4. Avoiding gratuitous harm and unnecessary risk

These goals have been listed here in what has conventionally, at least in the United States, been considered their usual order of importance. All health care professionals today are deeply committed to some version of these primary goals of health care for their patients. The items may differ in number, emphasis or ranking, depending on a variety of considerations that include: (a) the particular health care profession studied, (b) the particular health care professional's own hierarchy of values and (c) the exigencies peculiar to the particular case at hand. Still, the obligations of clinicians to patients and the principles that express those obligations are ordinarily construed in terms of concerns such as these.

Unfortunately, the first two of these goals are precluded by this man's pathophysiology. That is, neither a cure nor an alleviation of symptoms is possible and, since the patient is not conscious, he cannot have pain. The third goal is precluded except for minimizing loss of function; but, since this man's only functions are vegetative, it is debatable whether the language of goals and values can continue to convey anything more than a symbolic connection with this patient's situation. Lastly, what is supposed to count as "harm" and "risk" to patients in vegetative states is even less clear.

Since little has been gleaned from the above-mentioned goals and values that ordinarily assist health care teams in determining how to care for their patients, a proponent of an "applications" approach would counsel the health care team to appeal directly to the ethical principles informing these goals and values, i.e., autonomy, beneficence, non-maleficence and justice. Because the patient is indigent, he will be afforded, at least in principle, all of the same treatment alternatives that federal, state and local support makes available to any indigent patient within the community. Therefore, under a standard analysis of an individual case such as this, the health care team's concerns about justice are ordinarily limited to assuring that similar cases be treated similarly, i.e., that all of the social support mechanisms customarily available to patients in similar circumstances have been solicited and utilized.

This patient's persistent vegetative state renders him incapable of making his own treatment decisions. Because this patient has left no advance directives of any sort, the health care team has no way of ascertaining how he would now wish to be treated. Since the patient is incapable of either direct or indirect self-determination, the relevance of the principle of autonomy to this particular case is limited to mandating that respect for this patient obligates the health care team's participation in making treatment decisions for this patient. While a request for a court-appointed legal guardian would satisfy the team's legal obligations to the patient, it does not eliminate their ethical responsibilities. That is, even with a legal guardian designated to make treatment decisions, the health care team is still ethically accountable for whatever treatment (or non-treatment) they ultimately provide.

Thus, advocates of a principlist approach would claim that the principles of beneficence and non-maleficence are the ones central to the solution of this particular case. Yet, these principles offer no means for deciding whether beneficence and non-maleficence are best expressed by continuing or discontinuing this patient's life-sustaining treatment. In the final analysis, no matter how carefully the case is examined and weighed, these principles often end up serving only as *post hoc* rationalizations for the health care team's conflicting intuitions as to what might count (or, alternatively, if anything even can count) as "beneficial" or "burdensome" care for a patient limited to a vegetative existence.

The push, of course, is for closure. The health care team is committed to solving the immediate problem that confronts them: identifying and meeting their ethical obligations to this particular patient. A plan of care was, with considerable discussion, finally crafted for the patient in this case. After consultation with the hospital ethicist, the health care team concluded that life-extending treatment offered the patient no benefit.

The health care team requested that a legal guardian be assigned to the patient, be informed of the patient's situation and asked, as the patient's legal representative, to give permission for withdrawal of life-extending medical treatment. The guardian assigned by the court concurred with the position of the clinicians and granted permission to withdraw all medical treatment except for comfort measures. Subsequent to the removal of the ventilator, the patient's respirations and heartbeat became erratic. Within minutes the patient's own spontaneous respirations and heart beat ceased. The patient's eyes became fixed and dilated, and he was pronounced dead.

Because there was no way of ascertaining what this patient's wishes might have been, the health care team and legal guardian defended this decision to withhold treatment as the one that best reflected their concern and respect for this patient and his situation. They were agreed that since even delaying the decision-making process is a decision to do something, whatever decision was made would, in fact, constitute an act of substituted judgment. Respecting this patient entailed careful evaluation of the alternatives in terms of their fidelity to the general obligation of the health care professionals to practice non-maleficence and beneficence towards patients by choosing the alternative most consistent with the values and ideals that society has tacitly endorsed and patients have come to expect health care professionals to support and protect. Both the clinicians and the legal guardian defended withdrawal of life-extending treatment by arguing that it has been their experience that most persons having the opportunity to decide this issue in advance for themselves would not choose to be sustained in a vegetative state.

4.2 Medical Treatment For A Social Ill

A frail, elderly man without relatives or visitors has lived in an extended care facility for the past five years. While needing physical assistance with daily activities, such as bathing and walking, he is oriented to time and place. With increasing frequency over the past two years the following pattern of behavior is observed: the patient abruptly informs his health care providers that he will no longer take fluids or food because he wants to die.

Within several days, the man becomes semi-comatose and is sent to the nearest emergency room where he is re-hydrated by means of intravenous fluids and/or naso-gastric intubation. Upon recovery, he consistently expresses regret that he is still alive and disappointment with his caretakers for having over-ridden his wishes. The patient temporarily resumes adequate consumption of fluids and food, only to repeat the cycle in a few months' time.

4.2.1 Analysis

Assessment of this case requires a very careful medical work-up to rule out any endogenous depression, i.e., depression caused by organic processes that may be causing or exacerbating this patient's behavior. Even the most minor physical symptom, if it becomes chronic, can cause patients to become frustrated and depressed enough to have periods of hopelessness. Only after the health care team is assured that there is, to the best of their knowledge, no underlying biological or chemical origin for such behavior can their analysis be extended so as to tease out the psychological and social factors in the case.

Next, the psychological aspects of this case must be ascertained. The health care team needs to make a careful assessment of the patient's mental status, in both his compliant and non-compliant periods. This assessment should include both passively observing the patient's behavior and actively interviewing the patient to elicit his perceptions about his situation. It is crucial for the health care team to ascertain whether the patient understands and can explain his situation and his conflicting behavior patterns, including the fit between his intentions and his actions and the relationship between his actions and their likely consequences. In other words, he must be able to provide coherent reasons for his intentions and in defense of his actions.

Such an assessment is necessary to determine whether this man has "decisional capacity," the term currently being used in the fields of health care and health care ethics to describe the ability of persons to make autonomous choices about treatment alternatives. While there are a number of ways it has been described,[12] decisional capacity standardly includes these five criteria:

1. *Understanding*: the patient must be able to comprehend and discuss with a reasonable amount of coherence the relevance of the information that has been disclosed by the health care professionals
2. *Rationality*: the patient must be capable of reasoning appropriately about means and ends (i.e., goals)—the patient should be able to anticipate the probable consequences of choices or actions and, in contemplating an end or goal, should be able to indicate realistic ways in which it might be reached
3. *Space*: when time permits, the patient must be given sufficient opportunity and time for deliberation to the fullest extent possible
4. *Absence from coercion*: the patient must be protected, as far as possible, from internal forms of coercion (e.g., pain, faulty processing of information) and external forms of coercion (e.g., economic pressure, intolerable environmental conditions, etc.)
5. *Authenticity*: the values and world-view invoked by the patient to explain present decisions and behavior should be reasonably consistent with the values and world-view held by the patient in the past and, if not, rather convincing evidence of why such a shift has occurred should be present

To the degree that these five criteria are met, patients are considered capable of making autonomous decisions about their health care. That is why one of the most important—though, at times, quite subtle—assessments clinicians make in each and every medical encounter is an assessment of a patient's decisional capacity. In those patients considered to have decisional capacity, the principle of autonomy requires clinicians to respect a patient's right to make his or her own personal health care decisions, irrespective of whether the health care team agree with the particular decision in question. Parenthetically, it is important to note, here, that decisional capacity is not the same as legal competence. "Competence" is a technical legal term and is best reserved for its technical legal meaning. That is to say, that by law, all persons who are twenty-one or older (or who have demonstrated to the court that they have reached the age of reason) are presumed competent unless formally and specifically adjudged otherwise.

From the dialogue that inevitably occurs between the health care team and this particular patient in the course of his care, it should be possible for the caregivers to elicit from the patient a coherent account of his behavior and expectations. This account should clarify whether he understands the logical relationship between his actions and their likely consequences. The patient's past records should be reviewed for insights into the possible reasons for his conflicting sets of behavior patterns. For example, has anyone ever previously asked the patient about his views concerning death, what his life plans and goals both are and were, and how he relates these to each other? Perhaps it is not so much that he wants to die as that he simply does not want to continue to live in this manner.

In addition, the health care team should investigate whether the patient has exhibited a chronic or intermittent fixation concerning loss of control over his life, a fixation that may render him unable to make a realistic assessment of his actual over-all situation. Perhaps he feels disenfranchised and abandoned by his community—not an unreasonable or unjustified observation, given the way the frail and elderly in our society are often treated.[13] Does the patient interact thoughtfully and coherently with his environment? Does he have any sustained relationships with anyone at the facility? These are the kinds of questions that must be asked and answered as thoroughly as possible in order to ascertain (1) a realistic assessment of what the patient's situation is and (2) whether the patient adequately understands his situation and is capable of making autonomous choices regarding his health care.

In this particular case the health care team requested a psychiatric consultation. The psychologist found that the patient demonstrated a clear understanding of the implications of his refusal to take food or fluids in both his compliant and non-compliant phases. His reasons for taking these actions remained consistent in both phases: he had outlived all of his friends and family, and no longer had any outside interests. The patient felt that, while he had lived a very full and active life, he now experienced no personal or vicarious joys, had no satisfaction in his continued existence and was unable to accept the extent of his dependence on his care-givers. He had, in sum, nothing of value to live for and, unwilling to accept such a life of dependency, preferred that his life be over.

When asked why he would return to a compliant stage after his bouts of rejecting food and fluids, he replied that the need to battle his caregivers was such hard work that he needed time to regain his strength. In other words, his compliant phases were not evidence of inconsistency in his understanding or his reasons for acting as he had. The psychologist concluded that, in spite of the fact that the patient's behavior seemed to be exacerbated by an exogenous depression (a depression that is caused by factors external to the patient), there was no indication that this patient's capacity to make decisions was impaired.

A factor that weighs heavily in any psychiatric evaluation is the realization that, as in this patient's case, being depressed does not automatically render a person incapable of making rational decisions. There are circumstances in which depression is a most reasonable emotional response, so much so that its lack might actually be construed as an inappropriate or unreasonable emotional response.

The social aspects of the case are fairly straightforward on the standard approach. This man claims no family or friends and no social or religious affiliations. He receives minimal social security benefits and resides in a typical state-run extended care facility. While he participates in the activities that occur at the facility, he does so indifferently, as though fulfilling empty requirements. He is distantly polite, but remains firm in his rejection of all attempts to persuade him to give up his desire to end his life. But we will see that this is, at best, a superficial account of what is socially significant here.

The members of the health care team have, in this case, a commitment to a view of the patient's good that appears to differ significantly from the patient's.[14] This occurs because health care professions place a very high value on preserving life in our society. They are committed to offering life-extending treatment to patients who are not terminally ill and, thus, come to equate such treatment with acting from the principles of beneficence and non-maleficence. Therefore, a patient who demonstrates clear evidence of decisional capacity while persisting in what health care professionals see as self-destructive behavior can be exceedingly frustrating for them.

Unfortunately, to continue rescuing this patient from his own behavior while failing to change his underlying rationale for that behavior will only compound the problem since, in addition to being frustrating and futile, it actually increases this patient's physical and mental distress. This mismatch has not been adequately addressed—either by the standard approach to health care ethics or by the ethics of the health care professions. One primary source of the mismatch in this case lies in a difference of emphasis or focus concerning the meaning that "life" has for the health care team and the patient respectively, a topic that will receive more detailed analysis in chapter four.

Generally speaking, however, the health care team's focus is on life as a means to an end, as a necessary condition for the possibility of anything else.

But as a necessary means to every possible end, life so understood can appear to have an absolute value. Consequently, it is all too often the case that, an underlying, unstated and unrecognized assumption by clinicians develops—viz., that, irrespective of the quality of a particular patient's life, life must always treated as an end in itself and, thus, as desirable by all rational patients. From this perspective, choosing not to continue living is construed as irrational (and yet the health care team's persistence in supporting the patient's *life* instead of the *patient* is construed as rational).

In other words, the four primary goals of health care professionals mentioned earlier in the first case of this chapter, as well as the principles that direct them, are considered life affirming and, thus, all efforts in support of patients are seen as directed towards sustaining life. In this case, however, the patient has repeatedly demonstrated his rejection of life as inherently valuable. He finds it both counterproductive and irrational to pursue—or to be forced to pursue—its continuance. He has not, in fact, lost sight of his life as a means, but considers it to be a means that not only no longer serves his ends, but also actually frustrates them. It is possible that his caregivers might help him to see value in continuing to live, i.e., to see valuable ends to which his life is a means. But, should such efforts fail, the mismatch between his views and the health care team's response to the standard views of their professional obligations will persist.

Another source of frustration for the health care team lies in their recognition of the causal connection between this patient's sustained rejection of his current existence and the social conditions contributing to the quality of that existence. That is, our society's economic commitments to the elderly have tended to be grudging, at best. As a result, sustained attempts by our culture to include, as active and valued members of the community, elderly who are no longer completely self-sufficient, remain half-hearted and ineffectual. As with the previous case discussed, the caregivers involved with this man's case are concerned to provide this patient with care that is equitable to other patients in similar circumstances. But, since elderly patients in these circumstances are frequently sent to nursing homes that, in one degree or another, effectively remove them from societal interactions, the principle of justice, as standardly conceived, offers little solace for patient or clinician alike. Here, one might say that, while the principle of justice is formally recognized, there are, as it were, no "habits" in place—no institutional structures, no familiar patterns of practice, no recognizable means—for its effective realization.

In addition, even when health care professionals are sensitive to this connection, the prevailing view of the profession's obligations to patients is silent concerning what, if anything, they can or should do to address this issue. As a result, the health care team can come to feel as though they have been thrust into the position of fulfilling the tacit, formal requirements the health care institution promises the public without having access to the most reasonably effective means of doing so. One such means might be a political voice that can bear witness to the adverse effects that seemingly isolated and unrelated social conditions have on the health and lives of all individuals, but especially the weak, poor and elderly. But this is not something ordinarily considered ethically binding for health care professionals.

Furthermore, each of these four patient-centered goals can represent an expression of sensitive caring. Yet there are conflicting interpretations about their meanings and relevance for any given individual, especially in light of the psychosocial realities of this patient's life. As a result, any one of these goals, when assumed without the participation or approval of a patient who has decisional capacity, can result in that patient being treated merely as means to ends that, in reality, no longer include him.

This is a most inexcusable form of paternalism, irrespective of whether it is motivated from the principles of beneficence or non-maleficence or not. Hence, pursuing any of these goals as values removed from the patient's psychosocial reality—or appealing to any of the principles that guide us in understanding these goals as if they were isolated and *a priori*—without discussing what, in each particular case, counts as good reasons in favor of their support is worse than meaningless. Doing so prevents patients who have some degree of decisional capacity from participating to the degree that they are able in decisions about their own situation. This would, in effect, cause the health care team to violate the autonomy principle in the name of benevolence. As a result, actions that clinicians construe as flowing from the principles of beneficence and non-maleficence can actually promote or increase, rather than ameliorate, a patient's suffering.

Once again, it is my thesis that such mis-matches and gaps in analysis derive from the inadequacy of the concept of personhood and relationship presupposed by the standard approach. In this particular case, the health care professionals decided that, since the patient was not terminally ill, the principles of beneficence and non-maleficence prevented them from passively acquiescing to his wishes to be allowed to die by refusing fluids and food. They are left with the alternative of continuing to send this patient, when he becomes unstable and semi-comatose, to the emergency room, to be aggressively treated for his self-induced dehydration and starvation.

4.3 Hyperacute Rejection Syndrome

During an otherwise unremarkable pregnancy, a 26 year old woman developed myocarditis, a severely damaging inflammation of the heart which interferes with the ability of the heart to pump blood efficiently.

Although she eventually delivered a premature but viable and healthy infant, the patient's own cardiac function deteriorated to the point where a transplant was the only remaining chance for saving her life. After delivery, a properly matched donor heart eventually became available and she underwent a transplantation that involved no immediate complications.

Several hours post-transplant and while she was still in the recovery room, the patient's cardiac function rapidly began to deteriorate. It was apparent that she was experiencing a "hyperacute rejection" (a process of organ transplant rejection whose etiology is poorly understood and which in about 95% of cases leads to repeat rejection should another transplant be attempted). The patient was placed on mechanical pump support as the newly transplanted heart could no longer provide the pumping action required to keep the patient alive. While she is currently awake, able to speak and rational, the mechanical pump is, at its present stage of technological development, only a stop-gap measure. Therefore, if this patient does not receive another heart transplant, she will die.

When a heart that is a good match for this patient finally becomes available, it also happens to be an equally good match for another potential recipient who is awaiting transplant for the first time. The hospital ethics committee is asked whether the transplant team should re-transplant this patient or give the heart to the other waiting candidate.

4.3.1 Analysis

Some of the biological facts of this case are quite clear in their implications. This young woman will die unless a second transplant is attempted. In addition, since her first transplant failed because of hyperacute rejection, the likelihood that she will reject the second attempt is 95%. The current rejection rate for heart transplants on a first attempt is approximately 5-8%. Therefore, if the other waiting candidate is given priority, there is a significant increase in the probability that the salvaged heart will not be rejected.

Unfortunately, an important biological aspect of the case remains problematic. Hyperacute rejection is a syndrome that can be neither prevented nor, given the current state of the art, corrected after it occurs. Moreover, there is no way of anticipating which particular patients are at a greater risk for developing this syndrome. In other words, while statistics can offer valid inferences about the characteristics of a group of persons on the basis of numerical information obtained from a randomly selected sample of the group (i.e., the inference is from sample to larger population group), it cannot be used in reverse to identify *which* individuals within the population group exhibit the characteristics in question. Therefore, since patients prone to hyperacute rejection syndrome cannot be identified in advance, the syndrome cannot be used prospectively either to disqualify certain potential transplant recipients or to modify their ranking on the waiting list.

In addition to the other pertinent psychological aspects of this case, one would especially want to know precisely what the patient and her family and/or significant others had been told pre-operatively about transplantation and its possible complications. One would want to know, that is, whether there had been adequate discussion about the dismal prospects of surviving hyperacute rejection syndrome should it occur, and about the conditions under which re-transplantation would or would not be considered as an option. One would also want to know the patient's response to this information and her understanding of its implications. In addition, while this patient is currently presumed to have decisional capacity, the health care team or teams involved need to elicit from the patient just what that understanding amounts to for her, from her particular perspective.[15]

The main social aspects of the case are three-fold and concern the relationships between (1) the patient and the larger community, (2) the patient and the health care professionals who are her current caregivers and (3) the community and the caregivers. As far as the first relationship is concerned, the very existence of the national transplant program and all of the various social institutions connected with it clearly imply a *de facto* commitment on the part of the larger community to the quality of the lives of its individual members as potential transplant recipients.

Similar to the commitment of health care professionals to patients (as expressed in their respective codes of ethics), this commitment of the community to its members is governed by the principles of beneficence and non-maleficence.[16] However, along with this commitment come utilitarian considerations of distribution that may directly conflict with particular patients' best interests as well as the health care professionals' obligations to patients. Hence, these considerations can place the principles of autonomy, beneficence and/or non-maleficence in direct conflict with the principle of justice.

For example, for the transplant team to deny re-transplantation to this patient—assuming she would want to be re-transplanted—and to transplant the other potential recipient would clearly provide the greatest possibility of a successful organ transplant and, hence, increase the likelihood that the salvaged heart will not be rejected. However, this is something that clinicians find extremely discomfiting in their relationships with their patients, since denying re-transplantation to the first patient will directly result in her death, no matter who else might be saved. Hence, it should be an important part of the obligation of the community to its members—potential patients and health care professionals alike—to address the need for very explicit criteria in order to maximize equitable distribution of salvaged organs.

As far as the second relationship, the one between patient and health care professional, is concerned, though the health care team does have a relationship with other potential recipients, it differs from their relationship with this patient whose death, without re-transplantation is both imminent and certain. The death of the operated patient will predictably occur within hours; the death of the waiting recipient might be anywhere from a few hours to days, weeks, or possibly even months. While the death of both is certain, the recent transplant patient's is more imminent because the potential recipient's own heart is still functioning, albeit poorly. Hence, given the prevailing view of the special obligations generated by the patient/clinician relationship and a lack of institutional guidelines concerning re-transplantation in patients who develop hyperacute rejection syndrome, the transplant team will understandably see itself as having little choice but to offer re-transplantation to the patient whose first transplant has failed.

Yet, at the same time, under the prevailing view of the clinicians' obligations to patients, the mere acceptance of a patient as a candidate for transplant automatically establishes a patient/clinician relationship. As discussed previously, this relationship traditionally entails a wholehearted commitment on the part of clinicians to embark upon a course of therapy most beneficial for that particular patient. This includes maximizing that patient's medical good in terms that can—as much as possible—be understood, identified with and accepted by the patient. Therefore, once a health care team embarks along a course of therapy for a patient under their care, the patient expects this commitment to be whole-hearted and within the customary framework of what is available to all patients under similar circumstances.

Considering their bleak prognoses, it arguably would be more rational simply not to make re-transplantation an available option to patients who develop hyperacute rejection syndrome. However, for health care clinicians to make this determination on a one-to-one basis at the bedside would utterly transform the tacit but, nonetheless, deep and abiding therapeutic relationship of trust that has developed between patients and clinicians under the prevailing view of patient/clinician relationship. This is why "rationing at the bedside"—the practice of making clinicians responsible for resource allocation at the bedside on a case-by-case basis—is considered by many working in the field of health care to be both therapeutically and ethically suspect. That is, when the community asks clinicians to adhere to protocols that, in effect, disadvantage some of their patients to the advantage of others, it is asking these caregivers to act in ways that place them squarely at cross-purposes with the commitments, values and principles they have traditionally been asked to honor towards their patients.

As far as the third relationship is concerned, the one between health care professionals and community, it is also a relationship of tacitly understood *mutual* obligations. On the one side, health care professionals are obligated to the community in several senses. First, the training and practice environments of clinicians exist, and are supported and encouraged by public institutions and the pooled resources of the community—a substantial portion of which simply cannot be measured *solely* in economic terms. Second, health care professions are licensed by the community—i.e., given certain unique privileges earned by virtue of their demonstrated expertise—to engage in practices that are restricted to them alone. On the other side, the community, in turn, is obligated to these professionals who, because of their specialized training, are able to improve the over-all quality of the community through education, research and their ability to provide increasingly more sophisticated levels of care to patients. Thus, it would constitute a serious abdication of responsibility on the part of a community to expect clinicians to make allocation decisions *between* patients (traditionally a communal responsibility—at least in democracies) in addition to preserving their traditional commitments to each patient with whom they have a professional relationship. To expect clinicians to assume both of these conflicting obligations *simultaneously* is psychosocially damaging in the extreme, as it erodes trust, one of the primary "social lubricants" that make relationships and the development of robust individuals possible.[17]

The hallmark of an ethical problem is that, irrespective of what choice is actively or passively undertaken, some incommensurable good—be it principle, interest, ideal or value—is irretrievably lost. The problem is not that we don't *know* or haven't *discovered* what is "True," "Right" and "Good." Ethics is not about choosing between truth and falsity, right and wrong or good and bad—no one of even minimal intelligence would willingly make choices that are false, wrong or bad! An ethical quandary is marked by the realization that, no matter how one looks at a particular problem, there is no way to reconcile all of the competing values (goods, rights, truth)—there simply is no absolute or intrinsically good solution. Rather, there is a number of less than satisfactory alternatives, ranging from bad to worse—and *this* is the reality within which ethical discourse and decision-making must occur.

Still, there are better and worse ways of identifying the implicit features of an ethical problem so that a particular choice or action might, at least, be more accurately drawn and compellingly defended as the least ethically objectionable and, thus, preferred alternative. However, because it relies on the algorithmic application of principles that, in turn, presuppose conflicting visions of what it is to be a person, the standard approach is incapable of offering a persuasive alternative. To succeed and, at the same time, remain internally consistent, it would have to appeal to some widely recognized and accepted meta-principle, or set of meta-principles, in order to explain and/or justify how these principles are to be balanced when they conflict. The standard approach does not succeed in this respect.

ENDNOTES

1. T. Beauchamp and J. Childress, *Principles of Biomedical Ethics*, 4th ed. (New York: Oxford University Press), 1994.
2. Edmund D. Pellegrino and David C. Thomasma, *For the Patient's Good: The Restoration of Beneficence in Health Care* (New York: Oxford University Press), 1988.
3. Tom L. Beauchamp and James F. Childress, *Principles of Biomedical Ethics*, 3rd ed. (New York: Oxford University Press), 1989.
4. Warren T. Reich, ed., *Encyclopedia of Bioethics* (New York: The Free Press, 1978), s.v. "Ethics: Rules and Principles," by William David Solomon.
5. Earl E. Shelp, ed., *Beneficence in Health Care* (Dordrecht: Reidel), 1982.
6. For a summary of the five major conceptions of justice that are, at the end of the twentieth century, still open to debate, see Warren T. Reich, ed., *Encyclopedia of Bioethics: Revised Edition* (New York: Simon and Schuster Macmillan, 1995), s.v. "Justice," by James P. Sterba.
7. Immanuel Kant, *Groundwork of the Metaphysics of Morals*. Trans. and ed. by H. J. Paton (New York: Harper and Row, 1956), p. 106.
8. Glen C. Graber and David C. Thomasma in *Theory and Practice in Medical Ethics* (New York: Continuum, 1989), pp. 9-11.
9. For a discussion of a representative collection of models for relating normative theory to practice, see Warren T. Reich, ed., *Encyclopedia of Bioethics: Revised Edition* (New York: Simon and Schuster Macmillan, 1995), s.v. "Ethics: Normative Ethical Theories," by W. David Solomon.
10. John Dewey, *Logic: The Theory of Inquiry*, *LW* 12:108.
11. This case, which is analysed in Erich H. Loewy's *Textbook of Health Care Ethics* (New York: Plenum Publishing Company, 1996) is used with the author's permission. The analysis of the case as it appears in this chapter is my own.
12. In the ethics literature there is no consensus, as yet, on precisely what constitutes decisional capacity, and unfortunately, the terms "competence" and "decisional capacity" are often still used interchangeably. For an interesting discussion about capacity, see A.E. Buchanan and D.W. Brock's *Deciding for Others: The Ethics of Surrogate Decision Making*, (NY: Cambridge University Press, 1990), p. 18. For an alternative, though somewhat similar set of criteria for decisional capacity, see David T. Ozar and David J. Sokol's *Dental Ethics At Chairside: Professional Principles and Practical Applications* (St. Louis: Mosby-Year Book, Inc., 1994), p. 106ff.
13. Tom Ricketts, "How to Make the Poor Die Elsewhere," *The Washington Monthly*, February, 1983, p.43.

14. For a very interesting and thorough analysis of the various, and sometimes conflicting perspectives with regard to what constitutes the "good" of the patient, see E.D. Pellegrino and D.C. Thomasma, *For the Patient's Good: The Restoration of Beneficence in Health Care*, (NY: Oxford University Press, 1988), esp. chap. 6.
15. N.B.: A set of criteria for evaluating a person's decisional capacity can be found on page 37 of this chapter.
16. The pre-existent status of these principles is explained and/or justified according to standard approaches by regarding them either as laws of nature or as the result of social contract. As the first section of this chapter suggests, there are alternative ways of regarding principles, their status and how they function. Chapter four offers such an alternative account.
17. Both the term, "social lubricant" and the notion that trust is one of the necessary conditions for the possibility of social co-operation as well as robust individuality are derived from discussions with and various writings of Erich H. Loewy.

Chapter 3

Dewey's Methodology, Purpose and Central Assumptions

1. INTRODUCTION

In numerous writings and lectures throughout his long career, Dewey addressed what he considered to be the central problem of modern life, i.e., finding a way to restore the integration and co-operation between man's beliefs about the world in which he lives and his beliefs about values and purposes that should direct his conduct.[1, 2] Dewey was convinced that no headway will be made in addressing this central problem until creative intelligence replaces dogma in the vital task of resolving problems (whether they have been labelled "moral" or "scientific") that confront individuals in their daily lives.

For Dewey creative intelligence is both the process and product of reflective inquiry, an unending and dynamic process that is a central characteristic of sentient beings and the *sine qua non* of intelligent behavior. To the degree that beings can use this process of reflective inquiry to understand their individual and collective interests and values, they are able to participate actively in the creation of new—and the modification of existing—interests and values as well as in the actualization of their interests and values in the rest of their lives. For Dewey this task is, in effect, the very purpose of philosophy.

Since Dewey's method of reflective inquiry and its assumptions are central to this inquiry, what is needed at this point is a description of his approach and some cogent remarks in its defense. To that end, this chapter will review the basic characteristics, aims and implications of Dewey's naturalistic and pragmatic theory of experience. The multi-perspectival, pluralistic approach that underlies Dewey's philosophical perspective will be defended here, not as something infallible, but as a most potent antidote against presuppositions standardly accepted in health care ethics that misdirect our understanding of experience in general and of relationships with other individuals in particular.

2. DEWEY'S METHODOLOGICAL PERSPECTIVE

Few philosophers have managed to combine theory and practice in their lives as successfully as did John Dewey.[3] Like the evolutionary philosophy he espoused, his own philosophical perspective grew from a kind of Kantian intuitionism through Hegelian idealism and into various stages of instrumentalism. It culminated in an empirical naturalism that emphasized reflective inquiry as the most effective mechanism for understanding and controlling the continuous and dynamic interreactions between our physical, biological, psychological and social environments.[4]

Dewey's alternative to the methodology used in traditional approaches in ethics is fairly straightforward. He argued that instead of constantly trying to find ready-made prescriptions or formulae to be internalized as habits and routinely applied to problematic social and ethical issues, we need to cultivate a more versatile characteristic of our intelligence. It is one that has been restricted, at least for the past few centuries, to the narrow, practical sphere we call science. The habit Dewey wants to see more widely acknowledged and whole-heartedly adopted when addressing *any* perplexing issues—whether they concern fields that are often narrowly designated "science" or the realm that is customarily treated separately as "morals"—is the critical and practical activity of reflective inquiry.[5]

Dewey was convinced that many of the ills that plague modern society are the result of denying or minimizing the engaged and practical nature of reasoning. Dewey's experimentalism was the result of his overwhelming need to see the world whole by constructing what he called a logic, that is, a method of effective inquiry, which would apply without abrupt breach of continuity to phenomena designated by both of these words [viz., "science" and "morals"].[6] In *Logic: The Theory of Inquiry*,[7] Dewey identified inquiry simply as the systematic and progressive determination of an indeterminate situation. He painstakingly described what he called the continuum of inquiry as the process by which beliefs and knowledge are acquired.[8] A rather radical thesis fundamental to his account was that logical forms accrue to a subject-matter when it is subjected to controlled inquiry. By this he did not mean simply that logical forms are revealed or discovered, but that these logical forms *originate* in the operations of inquiry.[9]

This has two very important implications. First, the continuum of inquiry is thoroughly pragmatic. For Dewey, this meant that the goal of inquiry—the search for truth—is neither a quest for certainty nor a search for knowledge of some timeless, ultimate reality that exists independent of our experiences or beliefs. Rather, the goal of inquiry is pragmatic in the sense that what we identify as a "true" set of statements or beliefs will depend on how well it helps us to understand experience and to guide further conduct. According to Dewey this means that consequences will function as the necessary tests of the validity of propositions "*provided* these consequences are operationally instituted and are such as to resolve the specific problem evoking the operations."[10] Second, every aspect of an indeterminate situation—means and ends or goals, meanings and values, intentions, perspectives and consequences—when subjected to reflective inquiry, undergoes an evolutionary development in the process of being converted into one that is "so determinate in its constituent distinctions and relations as to convert the elements of the original situation into a unified whole."[11]

Hence, when Dewey uses the term "consequences," he is not limiting its meaning to a product of a narrow and linear process, the arguably narrow perspective of which the consequentialistic approach to ethics is often accused. He is reminding us instead that every aspect of our actions and our reflections on them must constantly be considered in terms of its impact on every other aspect—and upon itself as well. In other words, this is not merely a linear, future-oriented or forward-looking perspective. Rather, because it is it is a dynamic process in which we, as reflective agents, actively participate, reflective inquiry not only reconstructs the problematic situation being reflected upon; it also reconstructs us—our past and present as well as our future.

A situation becomes indeterminate and, hence, ripe for reflective inquiry whenever any reflexive activity—whether personal habit or public practice—is, for any number of reasons, blocked, disrupted or fails to produce an expected result. Such an indeterminate situation then becomes problematic when our knowledge or understanding of it fails to correct or explain it. Our very recognition of a situation as "problematic" already entails a complex and dynamic process in which means, ends or goals and perspective are thrown into doubt. In other words, our awareness of a situation as problematic signals that reflective inquiry is already underway.

Moreover, how an indeterminate situation is envisioned as a problem determines not only what information will be considered relevant to it, but also what will be identified or ruled out as possible solutions to be tested and evaluated. Just as inquiry is occasioned by an indeterminate problematic situation, the elements of the problematic situation are progressively reconstituted and, ideally, made more determinate by inquiry. In short, understanding the world in which we live is a process of which we are a part, and any knowledge that we might gain comes from taking part in events in an intelligent—i.e., purposive rather than reflexive—way.

While the resolved or reconstructed situation solves a particular problem at hand, it also sets the stage for further inquiry. That is, it becomes not only a means to further ends-in-view, but also the source of a whole new set of interconnected problems. It is, in this sense, simultaneously an end or goal and a means. Recognizing the multifaceted and evolutionary nature of the elements that constitute our experience permits us to locate and understand situations and their solutions experientially, and not as arbitrarily and artificially isolated exercises unconnected to daily living. That is why if we are to understand more fully the uniqueness and power of Dewey's account of reflective inquiry it is helpful to examine his theory of experience.

3. DEWEY'S PRAGMATIC THEORY OF EXPERIENCE

One of the most frequent accusations levelled against Dewey by his critics was (and is) that his philosophy blurs rather than clarifies important distinctions that are traditionally respected by philosophers. But, unlike those who claim that philosophy is essentially the art of making fine, precise distinctions, Dewey insisted that, what ever else it is, philosophy is a "doing." That is, it is the means by which we attempt to use our intelligence to make sense of our existence, to see the world whole. As a matter of fact, Dewey agreed that precise distinctions and their analyses are an important part—but only *one* part—of that activity. That is why he constantly warned against the folly of allowing any distinction to assume the status of a settled belief *writ large*, so to speak, whereby the meaning of a distinction becomes isolated from the particular problematic situation which called it forth and in which it was originally addressed.

Dewey often criticized this common but subtle reification of distinctions, calling it "the" philosophic fallacy.[12] Dewey saw this reification as a by-product of the quest for knowledge of some ultimate reality independent of experience. Dewey rejected the metaphysical assumptions behind this quest insisting that, for us, the importance of distinctions, like any other statements or beliefs, lies in their usefulness for making sense of experience and for guiding choice and action in daily life. That some distinction "is the case" always involves contextual interpretation of the related aspects of the particular case within which the distinction is being made. Even the fact *that* inquirers might agree about a distinction remains ambiguous until the story of *how*, *where* and *why* they came to agree is articulated. In other words, the reification of distinctions blurs their usefulness to us.

Throughout his career, Dewey called for replacing the customary tradition that combines "atomistic particularism with respect to empirical material and Platonic *a priori* realism with respect to universals" with a naturalistic view in which "every experience in its direct occurrence is an interaction of environing conditions and an organism."[13] In other words, the world and our reflections upon it constitute, as it were, a unified field: the world and our understanding of it are not to be considered apart from one another since neither exists apart from the other for us. For Dewey, experience is not the isolatable product of an interaction between separate entities and objects. Nor is it an intersection between the subjective field of a perceiver and objective "facts" neutrally read off of nature. Rather, it is a continuous transactional process wherein perceiver and object are progressively re-constituted. There is nothing mysterious about this process. We not only presuppose it, we expect it and, at times, we specifically invoke it—as, for example, when we ask a person to tell us what she "sees" in the abstract designs of a Rorschach test or when scientists provide us with computer-enhanced photos of Jupiter.

As early as 1896, Dewey introduced his re-interpretation of the reflex arc, a concept foundational to the science of physiology.[14] Dewey saw in it a means of explaining the unity of experience in all of its complex diversity and generality. Because experience is actively undergone and not passively observed, the stimuli and responses within experience are not insulated one-way circuits. Rather, they reverberate in a multi-directional, responsive and reciprocal manner that modifies every aspect of, as well as everything that undergoes the experience. Dewey continued to build upon this basic notion. By 1938 he had provided in his massive work, *Logic: The Theory of Inquiry*, a detailed and systematic treatment of the dynamic commonalities of the reciprocal interactions which occur between all organisms and their environments—commonalities, by the way, that are necessary for the very possibility of developing the kind of individuation that persons consider to be a defining feature of sentience:

> Whatever else organic life is or is not, it is a process of activity that involves an environment. It is a transaction extending beyond the spatial limits of the organism. An organism does not live *in* an environment; it lives by means of an environment...the only source of restoration of energy. Not even a hibernating animal can live indefinitely upon itself.... The processes of living are enacted by the environment as truly as by the organism; for they *are* an integration.[15]

This description has even more significance for interactions between complex, sentient organisms than it has for interactions of primitive one-celled organisms. That is, the more complex the organism and/or the environment become, the greater the complexity and number of new and different dynamic interreactions that can possibly affect and be affected by the life of the organism:

> Indeed, living may be regarded as a continual rhythm of disequilibrations and recoveries of equilibrium. The "higher" the organism, the more serious become the disturbances and the more energetic (and often more prolonged) are the efforts necessary for its reestablishment [sic]. The state of disturbed equilibration constitutes *need.* The movement towards its restoration is search and exploration. The recovery is fulfilment [sic] or satisfaction.[16]

As it is described here, an organism's response to a stimulus is much more than just a mechanical application of some pre-established means necessary to some antecedently given end or goal. Rather, it is a complicated cascade of reciprocal readjustments by organism and environment to a series of mutually generated stimuli and responses. It is within the course of such dynamic interreactions that organisms and environments acquire stability and that organisms become progressively more individuated and potentially more self-aware.[17]

Just as primitive organisms, if they are to survive, must rapidly develop the ability to differentiate between self and non-self in the course of their interactions with their environments so, too, do more complex, sentient organisms, including human beings. Basic textbooks in human physiology and psychology detail the initial inability of neonates to recognize self from non-self either immunologically (biologically) or psychosocially. Individuation, first biological and then psychosocial, is a progressive, developmental affair that is intimately connected with actively experiencing an environment. A perspective that is based on this much richer, bio/psycho/social account confirms the distortion that can occur in inquiry when any element of this complex and dynamic integration is examined in static isolation from the environment in which it occurs. Literally speaking, that element will become mysterious and quite incomprehensible.

According to Dewey, bio/psycho/social integrity can be effectuated in two ways: blind impulse and intelligence.[18] To the degree that humans are sentient organisms, they are capable of choosing intelligence over blind impulse in order to advance their goals while continuing to maintain their bio/psycho/social integrity. That is, to the degree that they are self-aware and have memory, they are capable of engaging in sustained self-directed reason. They can make distinctions about relevant similarities and differences, and they can choose to form the habit of exercising creative intelligence—Dewey's word for a habit of responsive and responsible, reflective inquiry—instead of relying on blind impulse to maintain or to restore what Dewey calls "dynamic equilibration."[19]

4. SCIENCE AS A PARADIGM FOR METHODOLOGY

Most of Dewey's critics—and even some thinkers sympathetic to his agenda—misunderstand his wholesale endorsement of the scientific method for all inquiry. It was never Dewey's intention to reduce ethics, religion or any other humanistic enterprise to a science, if by science is meant *merely* a descriptive account of material change. On the contrary, Dewey rejected any dualistic assumptions that separate science and values. According to Dewey, science can exclude human interests and valuings no more readily than such fields as ethics and politics can exclude the inquiries commonly labelled scientific. And that is hardly science in the broader sense Dewey intended by this word.[20] Rather, Dewey's point in praising science was to emphasize the unprecedented successes possible in any field or endeavor when dogma and intolerance are replaced by reflective inquiry. For Dewey reflective inquiry, when intelligently pursued, requires simple curiosity and an open but distinctively critical attitude: a willingness to suspend belief and expectation and the patience to cultivate healthy doubt until evidence is accumulated. Such an attitude rejects, for example, the anti-intellectual temptation of "premature closure," the practice of making a too hasty assumption, the error of which is then compounded by the selective marshalling facts to confirm it.

According to Dewey ideas are exciting possibilities. They are the social products of intelligent and creative individuals who have been habituated to the process of reflective inquiry.[21] Hence, ideas—whether the ideas of science or the ideas connected to values—must never be treated as dogmas to be asserted; rather they are live hypotheses that are continually open to testing and manipulation. No matter how "settled" a belief or idea, it must always be potentially falsifiable and open to public scrutiny. Its very status as a settled belief is, after all, the result of its continuous reconfirmation in actual practice. Dewey believed that these features of reflective inquiry have been most consistently and successfully modeled in the collaborative efforts of scientific communities than by any other sustained human enterprise to which we might look for examples.

In other words, what Dewey referred to as real science—as opposed to mere technological production or the rote replication of the intellectual products of real science—succeeds because it embodies the public process of deliberate and critical, but always open-ended reflective inquiry. This process occurs from the very beginning of an indeterminate situation, where our unreflectively held valuings are challenged, and continues throughout the complex process of attempting to make that situation less indeterminate. This process includes identifying the indeterminate situation as a problem, theorizing about it and its possible resolutions and then testing and evaluating the most likely means for resolving it. According to Dewey, whenever we engage in real science we are employing precisely this meaning of reflective inquiry. When he calls for a "scientific treatment of morality" all Dewey is asking is that we assume this distinctive critical attitude of reflective inquiry towards all things—material and immaterial alike—which have developed value and meaning for us.[22]

Consequently, any account of morality that offers a single, unimpeachable system of evaluating ethically problematic situations will have effectively closed itself off to elements of experience that are needed if reflective inquiry into ethical issues is to take place. On Dewey's account this closure nearly always occurs because some distinction that has proven extremely valuable in a specific ethically problematic case or context in the past has been reified into a universal and unchangeable norm instead of being understood as one of many potentially valuable tools forged out of past fruitful inquiries. Like any tool, because of its empirical status, these distinctions are subject to critical reflection, open to modification and, thus, cannot be fixed or immutable.

For Dewey, reflective inquiry is also a dynamic social affair: it is, ideally, a democratic process designed to give meaning and value to our experiences. As an abstract social ideal, democracy has often been associated in contemporary American culture with a vision of the individual as a pre-existing entity standing over against community. That is not the sense of the term, "democratic," that is intended here. Rather, the term, "democratic," is used here to describe a process—and an attitude about that process—which is public, social and collaborative precisely because experience itself is public, social and collaborative.

And so, inquiry is democratic in three important respects. First, like science, inquiry actively builds both directly and indirectly on the results of the past experiences of many individuals. Hence, inquiry is public. Second, even though it is individual persons who carry on reflective inquiry, their individuality is the result of ongoing interreactions between a self-conscious entity and its environment (which includes other self-conscious entities). Thus, inquiry is social. Third, even though each person's experiences are of a world that is populated and shared by other persons, each person has a unique history that is distinctively brought to bear in reflecting upon any experience. Since life's experiences are so very interconnected, myriad and complex, each person's narrative of his experiences is a potentially valuable resource for others. Therefore, inquiry that is carried on by persons is much improved by collaboration.

In other words (mine, not Dewey's—though consistent with his intent), whether viewed as a body of accumulated wisdom or regarded as an ongoing process, reflective inquiry is carried on by self-reflective individuals dialogically. But it is a dialogue in the very broadest sense of that term. That is, it refers neither to a pattern of logical argumentation nor to a mere synthesis of two opposites, but rather to the kind of democratic and interdependent engagement that occurs when a community of individuals come together seeking resolutions to common problems. This community can be any group—scientists, politicians, the town hall, a family, a health care team. Such dialogue occurs whenever any number of individuals come together to listen to one another, and to address together whatever is problematic that they face together, in the attempt to understand each other's different perspectives and to modify their responses accordingly. This kind of living, evolutionary communicative engagement Dewey regards as the *sine qua non* of reflective inquiry.

Some might also want to construe reflective inquiry as a "dialogue" with oneself. Certainly this tendency is present in individualistically oriented societies like our own. However, Dewey would insist that this "internal dialogue" is dialogue only derivatively insofar as it depends on one's being able to represent an hypothetical "other" with which to rehearse for dialogue.[24] There is also a sense in which some might be tempted to say that the "dialogue" of reflective inquiry can occur between an individual and some inanimate object within that individual's experience—say, a textbook. Yet, this is simply an individual's response to a culturally constructed and understood stimulus framed and communicated in terms of meanings that are already publicly shared.

Because in both these instances there is a lack of mutual understanding and active engagement (to some degree or other) by all participants in the discussion, these two examples remain dialogues in a very attenuated and potentially misleading sense since the rest of the community is not actively participating. On the other hand, the activity of the physical scientist at her workbench *is* a dialogue in Dewey's sense insofar as she is able to elicit from the materials she is testing a falsifiable "response." That is, a response which can be publicly understood and duplicated, and to which she and others in the community can publicly respond in turn.

Accordingly, .genuine inquiry must meet the requirements of dialogue: (1) active engagement, (2) publicity, (3) an effort towards mutual understanding of and respect for differences, (4) openness to the inevitability of modification or change and (5) a willingness to allow ourselves, individually and collectively, to be led by the dynamic of the inquiry rather than by our own predetermined expectations and interests. As a deliberate and dynamic habit or practice in problem solving, reflective inquiry is social through and through and encompasses past, present and future. When Dewey considers moral inquiry, then, he associates these five characteristics with it as well, for then it is inquiry at its best; it is the richest activity of intelligence at work; it is—to use the word Dewey often used for the purpose—science.

Dewey's is a pluralistic philosophy that, in its characterization of the creative intelligence of individuals as a social process of deliberate, sustained and reflective inquiry, makes it possible to celebrate the diversity and difference in its participants as strengths rather than as weaknesses. Because his theory of inquiry rejects the alleged discontinuity between science and philosophy and emphasizes the multi-perspectival, pluralistic, fallibilistic and pragmatic character of creative intelligence wherever it operates, it is especially appropriate for addressing conflicts that arise in the field of health care. The present re-examination and critique of problematic patient/provider relationships and the effort to add to how they are described in the current health care literature presupposes and utilizes the central assumptions of Dewey's philosophical approach that have been explained here.

5. CONCLUDING REMARKS: THE RELEVANCE OF DEWEY'S APPROACH FOR THIS WORK

The approach adopted in this work is one that takes seriously Dewey's objections to the traditional philosophical approaches to the analysis of ethical problems in general and adapts his alternative philosophical methodology specifically to ethical issues in health care. It begins by accepting, right at the outset, the implications that follow from recognizing the actual situatedness of sentient, rational experience. While this approach appeals to many of the same principles, rules, goals, values and virtues as the traditional approaches, these concepts are informed by a different set of presuppositions about the nature of persons. This different set of presuppositions acknowledges the interdependence that characterizes persons by incorporating into all discussion and deliberation the dynamic and fluid interrelationships between the complex and evolving environmental, biological, psychological and social aspects of sentient, rational existence.

Within this alternative approach concepts such as autonomy—whether they are taken to be principles, values or virtues—have no *a priori* essence or standing. Rather, they are treated as encrypted generalizations culled from the distilled wisdom of past experiences—an individual's own and others—having, as yet, ambiguous meaning for the people involved and the particular situation at hand. They represent ways in which the meanings of similar problems in the past have been expressed and/or addressed. Like basic recipes, they are versatile tools that help us to produce novel creations and variations depending upon the ingredients at hand.

The approach espoused in this work is a process whereby differing perspectives concerning a situation are, through the interreactive communication of dialogue, sought out and encouraged. Each alternative is subjected to what Dewey referred to as "dramatic rehearsal," the equivalent of thought-experiments in science. In dramatic rehearsal the antecedents and consequents of an indeterminate situation are imaginatively envisioned from a number of different perspectives and critically examined so that the tentative conclusions obtained might be integrated into current communication and debate. Analogous to the improvement binocular vision offers over monocular vision, viewing a situation from more than one perspective makes accessible to us the requisite contrasts and comparisons needed in order to better assess the significance of the interrelationships with a given situational field.

This activity of comparison and contrast is, in turn, somewhat analogous to the movements one makes in bringing a microscope into focus: the barrel of the microscope is wheeled up and down in progressively smaller ranges until the specimen on a slide is brought into the sharpest possible focus. Similarly, as elements of the indeterminate situation are brought into focus—become, as it were, more determinate—tentative hypotheses are developed from the elements of the situation itself, alternative solutions are imaginatively tested and possible consequences compared and evaluated. As the process continues all of the elements of the situation are funded with meaning, including the principles of action that guide further responses to the situation and the consequences of its resolution. As a result, an indeterminate situation becomes progressively more determinate.

Thus, this alternative approach differs both in its emphasis on interdependence as a significant characteristic rather than a defect of persons and in its adoption of a method of inquiry that is better equipped to explain these dynamic interrelationships. Consistent with its emphasis on interdependence, this approach relies upon the provision of an environment that is conducive to communication and discussion, since it requires an opening, as it were, within which a meaningful story can develop out of a problematic situation that is fraught with indeterminacy. Before an assessment of this alternative approach can be undertaken, however, both the presuppositions about persons and relationships underlying the traditional approaches and the four principles that these presuppositions inform (namely, autonomy, beneficence, non-maleficence and justice), need to be reconstructed. That is the focus of chapter four.

ENDNOTES

1. John Dewey, "Experience, Knowledge and Value: A Rejoinder," *LW* 14:61-62.
2. Readers are reminded that during the period in which Dewey wrote (late 19th and early to mid-20th centuries) it was customary to substitute the term "man" for the terms "human being" and "human race." Hence it should not be assumed that Dewey's use of the term "man" or "men" (e.g., *Problems of Men* {*LW* 15:153-285}) was sexist or insensitive to the intelligence or interests of women. On the contrary, Dewey was one of the few philosophers to anticipate—and to welcome—the eventual involvement of women in philosophy. In the 1919 essay "Philosophy and Democracy," for example, Dewey wrote:
   > "Women have as yet made little contribution to philosophy. But when women who are not mere students of other persons' philosophy set out to write it, we cannot conceive that it will be the same in viewpoint or tenor as that composed from the standpoint of the different masculine experience of things." (MW 11:45)
3. Of his first four articles published, three introduced themes Dewey would spend the rest of his long career re-thinking and re-working, a process indicative of and consistent with the critical and evolutionary methodology he propounded. Dewey, "The Metaphysical Assumptions of Materialism," *EW* 1:3-8; "Knowledge and the Relativity of Feeling," *EW* 1:19-33; and "Kant and Philosophic Method," *EW* 1:34-47.
4. For a good *précis* of his professional development as a philosopher, see Dewey's essay, "From Absolutism to Experimentalism," *LW* 5:148-60. For an account of the evolution of Dewey's thought see, for example, Morton G. White, *The Origin of Dewey's Instrumentalism* (New York: Columbia University Press, 1943) or Richard J. Bernstein's chapter entitled *John Dewey* in the *Great American Thinkers Series* edited by Arthur W. Brown and Thomas S. Knight (New York: Washington Square Press], 1967), chap. 2.
5. Dewey objected to the polar distinction frequently drawn between science as the study of temporal and material change and morals as the study of timeless and changeless truths. While many of his works deal with the problems that such rigid distinctions create when assumed wholesale, prime examples of Dewey's treatment of this topic can be found in such essays as "From Absolutism to Experimentalism" (*LW* 5:147-60, esp. 156), "Philosophy" (*LW* 5:161-77), "What I Believe" (*LW* 5:267-78) and *Problems of Men* (*LW* 15:154-69). An example of his more extended treatment of the topic can be found in *Reconstruction in Philosophy* (*MW* 12:77-201).
6. *LW* 5:156-7.
7. Dewey, *Logic: The Theory of Inquiry*, *LW* 12.
8. Ibid., p. 16-7.
9. Ibid., p. 11.
10. Ibid., p. 4.
11. Ibid., p. 108.
12. Dewey, *MW* 14:123.

13. Dewey, "Experience, Knowledge and Value: A Rejoinder," *LW* 14:29.
14. Dewey, "The Reflex Arc Concept in Psychology," *EW* 5:97-109.
15. Dewey, *Logic: The Theory of Inquiry*, *LW* 12:32.
16. Ibid., p. 34.
17. For a more extensive review of Dewey's technical references to individuation see, *LW* 12: 74; 109; 125; 220; 238; 351; 441. The works most frequently cited concerning how his notion of individuation plays out in practice are *Human Nature and Conduct* (*MW* 14) and *Individualism: Old and New* (*LW* 5).
18. Dewey, *Human Nature and Conduct*, *MW* 14: Part III: "The Place of Intelligence in Conduct," pp.119-190, esp., pp. 175-8.
19. Ibid., pp. 125; 173.
20. Dewey denied that any field of scientific endeavor could be divorced from the interests, needs and purposes of those beings whose endeavor it is. See footnote #5 above, as well as his "Logical Conditions of a Scientific Treatment of Morality," *MW* 3:3-39.
21. Ibid., p. 124.
22. Dewey, "Logical Conditions of a Scientific Treatment of Morality," *MW* 3:3-39.
23. Dewey, *MW* 14: xi-xii; 16; 60-1; 96-7; 201-3.

Chapter 4

Re-assessing Some Traditional Presuppositions about Persons

1. OF PERSONS AND PATIENTS: CONCEPTS AND EXPERIENCE

While there are a number of ways in which ethical issues between patients and health care providers can be discussed and analysed, persons remain the primary unit of moral reference and, thus, the central feature of such discourse. The focus of this chapter is to examine some prevalent presuppositions about persons that shape and are shaped by the set of concepts (especially autonomy and beneficence, but indirectly non-maleficence and justice as well) that are relied upon so prominently in standard approaches to health care ethics analysis today.

The importance, ranking and use of these concepts—whether, for example, they are treated primarily as abstract principles or as concrete values—depends largely on the particular philosophical approach in question. But, irrespective of approach, the utilization of some variation of this set of concepts is central to most contemporary discussions, especially in health care ethics, concerning how to identify and to protect or to restore what are considered to be definitive characteristics of persons. By examining how these characteristics are expressed and reinforced in habitual behavior, our presuppositions about what it is to be a person can be identified and subjected to further inquiry. The next several sections discuss problems associated with conceptualizing these characteristics when the concepts used to do so are not fine-grained enough to do the work asked of them because of insufficiently critical presuppositions about persons upon which they are based. The perspectives explained in chapter three, drawn from the work of John Dewey, will be especially useful in unpacking the errors of these presuppositions and how they affect the standard health care ethics approach.

2. A CAUTION ABOUT CONCEPTS

A concept is generally construed as the product of an attempt to capture and to fix in an abstract and non-dynamic form certain generic aspects of a complex, concrete experience that is fluid and dynamic. When considered alone, bereft of context, this non-dynamic form can serve only as a placeholder. That is, it is but a reminder of the potential that an experience can have for a person, depending on antecedent conditions (which include the distilled wisdom learned from similar past experiences—our own, but especially that communicated to us by others), present context and the availability of the means necessary for realizing those possibilities.

Until the material conditions of the particular story or case it is connected with are identified, the meaning of a concept will retain a certain openness which gives it its characteristic ambiguity. When a situation is read in terms of some favored or pre-determined understanding of such a concept, that open range of possibilities can be prematurely closed and the possibility of a mismatch between concept and reality increases. When this happens, we may feel quite confident that our understanding of a situation has been improved when, in reality, it has actually become *more* rather than less indeterminate.

Concepts are important tools that can function very well as effective pieces of intellectual shorthand. However, it is possible for a concept, like any tool, to obfuscate as well as to clarify an already indeterminate situation. The meaning of any concept cannot be given once and for all because its context is never given once and for all. That is, the meaning of a concept changes as the bio/psycho/social field within which it functions and is framed changes. Whenever aspects of an existence that is inherently characterized by change are isolated and fixed by externally pre-established concepts—whether these have been formulated as principles, rules, criteria, values or virtues—there is an element of risk involved. These concepts can distort our understanding of an experience by artificially isolating and fixing upon certain aspects of an existence that is, in reality, both more complex and inherently characterized by change.

The difficulty is exacerbated if we allow ourselves to assume the adequacy of and to be guided by a single pre-interpreted perspective. This occurs when we attempt to make sense of unexpected hitches in our complex and evolving interrelationships, experiences that are marked by periods of disruption as well as periods of dynamic and homeostatic balance. To the degree that we uncritically accept and act from such a perspective we eliminate, without adequate reason, certain points of view and, in turn certain possible meanings of and alternative resolutions for an indeterminate situation. This is why what are today called "principlist" approaches—i.e., ones that analyse indeterminate situations by applying concepts externally pre-established from a particular pre-existing perspective—are so problematic. The discussion of health care ethics that issues from today's standard perspective, as exemplified in chapter two, suffers from just this problem.

3. THE MYTH OF THE INDEPENDENT AGENT

One of the central tenets of the standard approach to health care ethics being examined here is the belief that a person's autonomy is compromised by illness. This belief is based on the fact that, when functionally compromised by injury or illness, a person becomes more dependent on others. According to this approach, this reduction in a person's ordinary functioning is said to contribute to a reduction in her autonomy.

Now, it is fairly straightforward and uncontroversial that, as illness decreases a person's ability to function, it increases that person's dependence upon others. Unfortunately, what too often occurs within the standard approach is that dependence itself, rather than its relative increase or decrease, is set in opposition to autonomy. This reinforces a presumption that persons are not normally dependent but, rather, complete and self-contained entities that exist independently from the rest of their environment unless or until they become functionally compromised.

Closely connected to this presumption is the belief that, under ordinary conditions, individuals control whether and how their lives will affect and be affected by others. As a result, autonomy comes to be treated as the "default mode" of human existence and is defined in terms of atomistic isolation: persons are self-contained, self-sufficient, self-defining and completely self-determined. In this default mode, justice is represented primarily in negative terms, such as non-interference and non-maleficence; and any role that beneficence might have is limited to those exceptional circumstances when such an atomistic view of persons either has been or is in danger of being compromised. In short, autonomy is held in stark opposition to dependency of any sort and the co-operative interdependence required in actual living—if the autonomy that persons are actually capable of is to develop and flourish—is ignored.

But there is no such necessary one-to-one connection in real life between autonomy and independence. Respecting a person as an autonomous being actually requires taking into account an interdependence of the very sort ignored by this atomistic interpretation of autonomy. Interdependence need not be viewed as a defect, even when it is increased or modified as a result of illness or injury; it is already a fundamental fact of human existence. As Dewey put it:

> The idea of a natural individual in his isolation possessed of full-fledged wants, of energies to be expended according to his own volition, and of a ready-made faculty of foresight and prudent calculation is as much a fiction in psychology as the doctrine of the individual in possession of antecedent political rights is one in politics.[1]

In other words, a person does not exist in a ready-made state that can be disembedded from all context. A person participates in and evolves within a dynamic and continuous field of complex interreactions. Therefore, when the standard approach to health care ethics narrows its view of autonomy to total independence, it necessarily misses many important features of the issues it examines, as the re-examination of chapter two's cases in chapter five will make clear.

4. ZOE AND BIOS

In order to understand why the concepts we use to talk about persons are especially problematic—a difficulty that is widespread, but especially problematic for the standard approach—it will be helpful to look at our English word, "life." As it is used in English it is a particularly ambiguous concept because it does not distinguish between "being alive" and "having a life."[2] In Greek, there are two words, *zoe* and *bios*, used to refer to the concept known in English as "life." *Zoe* is life in a physiochemical sense, i.e., "being alive." *Zoe* provides the basis of our word, zoology, the biological science of animals.

Bios, on the other hand, is life in a bio/psycho/social sense, i.e., "having a life." *Bios* is the basis of our word, biography, a written history of a person.[3] *Bios* presupposes *zoe* insofar as to have a life, one must be alive. But *zoe* (being alive) does not guarantee *bios* (having a life), it merely provides the physiochemical substrate for its possibility. *Bios*—having a life—means being a reflective subject of a life. That is, having a life entails sufficient consciousness—at minimum, a rudimentary sentience and memory—to recognize self and environment, to appreciate how they are interconnected, and to effect a delicate balance of those interconnections through the ability to reason—even if quite rudimentarily—about means and ends or goals.

Persons, in addition to being alive, are also rightly said to possess that life. A person is the subject, the agent/patient as it were, of a particular life, with a particular history, within a particular dynamic and holistic set of environing conditions and experiences—environmental, biological, psychological and social. Persons actively undergo life in the sense of *bios*; because they are able to reflect upon experiences—both direct and vicarious ones—they can learn to modify experience as well as their responses to it by becoming active participants rather than merely passive recipients. This is why *bios* cannot be reduced to or explained solely in terms of *zoe*.

The implications of this distinction for health care are especially profound since the *zoe*-istic or physiochemical aspects of life cannot account for the role that the bio/psycho/social elements characteristic of having a life play in constituting persons. Without concepts in discourse that distinguish clearly between being alive and having a life, it is difficult to avoid a mechanistic view of persons and to adopt, instead, a holistic view of persons as reflective subjects of lives. A mechanistic view sees persons as discrete and self-contained objects merely reacting to other objects in their environment. In contrast, a holistic view sees persons as agent/patients who are constantly redefining and being redefined by their participation in a dynamic and homeostatic interrelationship with an environment. The term, "homeostasis," is used here to express the fluid and dynamic nature of both the elements that are interreacting and the activity of balancing those elements so as to optimize one's existence within and with an environment.

This failure of the standard approach to sufficiently distinguish between being alive and having a life also reinforces what, in the culture of the United States, is already an overly individualistic interpretation of persons. This, in turn, influences the way other concepts central to ethical discourse in health care are treated. In order to answer questions about what constitutes treating persons who are patients with respect, the features that must be taken into account and addressed regarding persons are not those belonging to *zoe*, but to *bios*. So, by adopting this distinction between having a life and being alive, we could more readily focus upon what is distinctive about persons and articulate a much richer understanding of the concepts associated with that distinctiveness.

Unfortunately, the standard approach to health care ethics today is as narrow in its conception of life as it is in its conception of autonomy/independence. The distinction articulated here in terms of *zoe* and *bios* plays little role in the analysis of cases according to the standard approach, as the examples in chapter two demonstrate. When these cases are re-examined in chapter five, the implications of distinguishing between being alive and having a life will be developed in more concrete detail. In the next section, an examination of John Dewey's analysis of organisms in relationship to their environments will contribute to this discussion.

5. AN ALTERNATIVE SET OF PRESUPPOSITIONS ABOUT PERSONS BASED ON THE CONCEPT OF BIOS

In his discussion of the reciprocal interaction between a living organism and its equally complex and dynamic environment, Dewey discusses how organisms become individuated. This explains why the integrity of the organism/environment interrelationship is a critical material condition for the integrity of the organism itself.[4] Such a holistic way of conceptualizing an organism not only emphasizes the elemental and dynamic homeostatic interrelationship between every organism—not only the human organism—and its environment. It also reflects how complexly and inextricably organisms—especially human organisms—are mutually bound to one another and to the environment they share. In fact, the interdependence between organism and environment is so profound that the organism is literally indefinable and incomprehensible when isolated from that environment:

> The processes of living are enacted by the environment as truly as by the organism; for they *are* an integration....[It is not simply] that a fish lives *in* the water and a bird *in* the air, but that the characteristic functions of these animals are what they are because of the special way in which water and air enter into their respective activities.[5]

Similarly, the characteristic functions of the intelligent organisms we call persons are what they are because of the special way in which environment enters into the activities of persons. On this account, what a person's basic needs and interests are and how they might be met are bio/psycho/social constructs insofar as they are a mutual evolution of organism and environment.[6] Persons, when considered in total isolation from the environment within which they pursue the activities connected to their having a life, are also quite literally indefinable and incomprehensible.

One implication of this evolutionary interrelationship is that it is profoundly irrational for persons, in the course of satisfying their own basic needs and interests, to act from the belief that they must consider themselves in opposition either to each other or to their environment. Both organism and environment mutually participate in and contribute to the determination of the organism's basic needs and interests. Thus, if individual persons are to flourish (i.e., if they are to have a life, if they are to have their basic needs and interests met, if they are to benefit from their participation in a part of a bio/psycho/social existence), their integrity cannot be purchased, either routinely or for very long, but only briefly and superficially, at the expense of disrupting the integrity of the rest of the environment of which they are a part. In this sense, it is quite correct to say that the progressive and continued flourishing of the individual entails the progressive and continued flourishing of the whole. The contrast between this conception of persons and that presupposed by the standard approach, especially in its appeals to its particular notion of autonomy, is significant.

Consequently, an important part of what it means for persons to maintain a homeostatic balance within an environment includes their realization that, in satisfying their needs and interests, they must do so in such a way that the integrity of the organism/environment interrelationship is respected. This presupposes that persons, as intelligent organisms, are capable of understanding and acting in a manner consistent with this fact, namely, that their own well-being and flourishing depends on preserving and enhancing the delicate balance of all organism/environment interrelationships. More specifically, since persons' needs and interests are so heavily influenced by and bound up with the social aspects of their environment, persons must understand that the satisfaction of their needs and interests depends upon, indeed can only be a consequence of, an irreducible and dynamic connection between individuals. The atomic individual idealized in the standard account of autonomy is simply a fiction and, when treated as reality, is capable of profoundly disrupting persons in their quest to meet their needs and interests.

Thus, for one person to have a life in any relevant sense (*bios*) requires the existence and involvement of others who can also recognize, value (even if only potentially or vicariously) and, in some situations, creatively participate in that life. No matter how self-directed or self-sufficient individuals do become, and ought to become in actualizing their potentialities, a whole community of others will have had, and will continue to have, a hand in both the development and the continued flourishing of every individual.

Moreover, it is important to understand here that it is not simply intimate personal others who have a hand in this activity. It is *all* others—including those never personally known to the individual—who publicly and privately participate in the creation of that complex community (which is made up myriad kinds of particular relationships, associations and communities) of others. That is, a community of persons is the function of persons interreacting with and by means of each other and their surrounding environment. The resulting characteristics of that community affect and are affected by every person's interreactions. In short, individuals need a complex, many-faceted nurturing community to help them develop their own unique capacities and talents. Likewise, communities, if they are to flourish and to interreact with individuals in this way need individuals who are motivated to reciprocate such nurturing and care in their own unique ways.

Thus Dewey's account of the reciprocal and dynamic interdependence that exists between organism and environment and his description of how that interdependence modifies the development and capacities of both organism and environment provides an alternative way of understanding ourselves as persons and of understanding, therefore, the nature of our obligations to one another. Each person has a unique biography; but it is one which others have played, and continue to play, an integral part in creating, nurturing and protecting. In other words, I am the person I am because of contributions others have made towards satisfying my basic needs and helping to develop my particular talents and interests. These contributions began long before I was capable of recognizing self from non-self and, if I am fortunate, will continue so long as I am capable of having an interest.

In addition, the satisfaction of basic needs and the assistance given me in developing my particular talents and interests are things I neither contracted for nor solicited from others—irrespective of whether I could or would have. The notion, so common in contemporary discussions of autonomy, that contract precedes social interaction is as much a fiction as that of the atomic individual. A significant portion of the conditions of my existence have been and continue to be outside of me and, yet, are also intimately bound up in my self-identity. That other persons routinely and without being expressly solicited have, for example, prevented or relieved my suffering from unmet basic needs is indicative of the fact that I am valued—for whatever diverse reasons. To the extent that I am who I am rests on the fact that I have been valued in this manner, I cannot even begin to describe myself in terms that exclude this fundamental interrelationship with others.

My understanding of myself and my expression of my own value may be distinguished from, but it cannot be separated from this complex bio/psycho/social interdependence between myself and my environment. To the degree that I am sentient and rational, these facts will therefore command my attention and demand an accounting, since a central feature of what it is to *be* sentient and rational is the ability to reflect critically about (i.e., to attempt to make sense of) one's situation. Another common fiction is that autonomous individuals reflect first alone and only later bring their reflections to others. But in point of fact, such reflection includes the process of asking and giving reasons—a process that itself presupposes community rather than isolation.

Moreover, it is only in comprehending my existential situation as one of fundamental interdependence that the origin and reciprocal character of such notions as debt, gratitude, trust, sympathy, empathy, commitment, responsibility and obligation begin to unfold and become determinate. This interdependence implies that obligation and, in turn, other concepts through which obligation is expressed (e.g., autonomy, beneficence, non-maleficence and justice) must be understood not as duties imposed on persons from without, but as intrinsic features of having a life. That is, interdependence and obligation are no different from any other concepts insofar as they are the attempts of persons to make explicit the meanings of the norms that are implicit in the social practices they participate in and within which they are already immersed.

These particular concepts are generated as a result of the myriad inferences persons make and tacitly share about their mutual situation. Because of the way in which they are generated, concepts cannot possibly have a meaningful existence outside of the "having" of a life, outside of an experience that is thoroughly bio/psycho/social. Concepts are neither derived nor imposed from without; they represent the explicit working out of what is already implicit in a dynamic and complexly evolving bio/psycho/social existence.

6. AUTONOMY AS A BIO/PSYCHO/SOCIAL CONCEPT

On this reconstructed view of persons, autonomy can no longer be viewed as the ideal independence of an isolated, individual self. Instead, our notions of self-rule, self-control, self-determination, self-governance, freedom, liberty, choice must all be taken to refer to an individual self that is neither simply a finished product of organism/environment interaction nor some disembedded, implacable and disinterested spectator but, in fact, a person that has unique and distinctive traits by reason of being an entity capable of intelligence and embedded in a dynamic organism/environment field in process. Autonomy, on this reconstructed view, comes to signify much the same thing as Dewey spoke of as "freedom":

> a *distinctive* way of behaving in conjunction and *connection* with other distinctive ways of acting, not a self-enclosed way of acting independent of everything else.[7]

It is simply impossible for the result of an individual person's proper growth and development to be "autonomous" in the sense presupposed by the standard approach, i.e., completely self-reliant and isolated from the influence of others. Rather, the stability and self-possession associated with the features so highly prized by persons as being a part of what they consider autonomy to be can, in fact, occur only within a particular kind of environment. It must be an environment of nurturing and care, a milieu characterized by the existence of already complex co-operative interrelationships and practices, both tacit and explicit, and both spontaneous collaborative activities and carefully organized and structured practices having a long history of development in their own right. None of our experiences and none of our reflections about them occur in a vacuum; they are always understood in terms of various relationships, associations, communities and, inevitably, cultural perspectives. Therefore, even when a person has an experience when no one else is present, her experiencing and her understanding of it are imbued with and filtered through communal frameworks. Hence, an obligation to respect a person's autonomy requires more than a formal, abstract recognition that individuals, by virtue of being persons, have a right to make their own decisions; i.e., ought to be, in some sense, left alone, unhampered. It also requires an appreciation of the role that a person's numerous connections to her community play in determining how effectively she will be able to realize that autonomy as, for example, in actualizing her capacity for decision-making.

This is why doing nothing more than formally recognizing the abstract legal rights of persons who have suffered, for example, racial or sexual discrimination is not simply ineffectual but often counterproductive. It is why concrete measures must also be introduced to redress inequities existing in both formal social institutions and informal social practices that have been ingrained by past insensitivities, as well as the long-term effects of these on the individual and collective psyches. It may be, relatively speaking, a straightforward process to change the policies of a political institution. It takes far longer to change the effects that the political enculturation of prior policies has had on the daily lives of persons, because such a change must address causal processes in the formation of persons, identities, concepts and behaviors that are far more complex, but just as important.

So, to respect formal autonomy without, for example, securing equitable access to the effective means of its realization—i.e., without making it a lived experience for all persons—fails to respect persons precisely because it ignores the interdependent play of bio/psycho/social antecedents and consequents that determines in actual practice what autonomy will effectively amount to for persons. Just as the ability to distinguish self from non-self emerges slowly as a person begins to experience having a life—thanks to, among other factors, the assistance and support of others who provide a safe space within which to develop and appreciate those experiences—so effectively expressing and maximally benefitting from genuinely autonomous behavior develops in the context of intelligent (i.e., critical and reflective) interreactions between persons. Obviously, a health care ethics—or a system of ethics of any sort—that is built on a concept of autonomy that ignores these realities about what it is to be a person will overlook much of ethical significance.

7. BENEFICENCE AND NON-MALEFICENCE AS BIO/PSYCHO/SOCIAL CONCEPTS

On the view espoused by the standard approach to health care ethics examined earlier in chapter two, beneficence and non-maleficence are regarded as principles that regulate conduct towards persons as isolated subjects deserving of "respect," a notion that, in turn, is based on an inexplicit and quite narrow intuition as to the characteristics of personhood. On the reconstructed view of persons as bio/psycho/social entities, beneficence and non-maleficence cannot be regarded simply as forms of substituted autonomy, with "autonomy" referring to the decisions and actions of isolated, individual selves. Something much richer and, in terms of obligations and relationships, something much more complex is needed. Empirical evidence clearly demonstrates that persons cannot begin to develop their individual talents and characters—much less contribute to or participate in a common life—without the beneficence and non-maleficence of others. But this is only to re-iterate that persons begin as completely helpless selves, unable to survive without a community of others willing and able to protect them from harm and suffering, to provide for their basic needs and to act as their mentors.[8]

Parenthetically, the term, "mentor," has specifically been chosen here as a contrast to the usual structured educative relationships in which teachers actively convey information that learners relatively passively absorb. Learning (both formal and informal) is too often viewed as a one-way process, from teacher to learner, and where the purpose of having the learner respond is primarily to verify that the information has been absorbed. But in such a process, students do not learn how to think but only, if anything, what to think—which is then treated as a set of facts or as the product of someone else's inquiries. In mentoring, as the term is used here, all parties are actively engaged; all contribute to the process, which is not confined to a particular time, place or structure.

Consequently, in mentoring everyone is both teacher and learner and, in the communication that results, *listening* becomes the quintessential feature of the process. Such "listening" involves more than simply a passive registering of isolated facts communicated by another. Rather, it requires of the listener the curiosity and imagination to set aside his own particular situation and perspective and to enter into the situation and perspective of the speaker, representing her perspective charitably and with as much fidelity as possible. A very important part of decision-making involves learning how to represent alternatives with charity and fidelity.

Even after persons have developed sufficiently to exhibit decisional capacity or, further, to be considered legally competent, they remain immersed and continue to participate in, by means of and with an environment that is interdependent through and through. Unless a person's life is suddenly and unexpectedly cut short, it is ordinarily the case that, as persons age, their dependence upon others—to help them meet those basic needs necessary for them to continue to carry out their routine daily affairs, to pursue their life plans and goals and to participate in and with the environment they share—will eventually, once again, increase.

But, perhaps most importantly, beneficence and non-maleficence can no longer be treated as attitudes and activities directed solely towards others. Certainly, this is not to deny the importance of being sensitive to or concerned about the good of others or their potential harm. Rather, it marks the fact that behaving beneficently or non-maleficently makes us feel alive and in control of our own lives: we are most likely to discover who we are—sometimes to our dismay—during those interreactions where our interests and concerns are directed towards others. This discovery is a characteristic feature of persons; it is one of the fulfillments of potential that, through critical reflection, self-assessment, and personal growth and development, persons are capable of realizing.

Since, as with any interreactions that involve persons, the responses of the social environment to a person's behavior will play an important role in the development of the person whose behavior it is, feedback (non-verbal as well as verbal) communicated by others will reinforce the development of attitudes and patterns of behavior that eventually come to characterize a person's unique sense of self. When guided by thoughtful and whole-hearted critical reflection, this feedback between persons (from intimates to complete strangers) constitutes a life-long, reciprocal mentoring process of listening, communication and growth, a process necessary for the perpetuation of persons as individuals who are members of various forms of community, a process not unlike Dewey's notion of democracy:

> that form of social organization, extending to all the areas and ways of living, in which the powers of individuals shall not be merely released from mechanical external constraint but shall be fed, sustained and directed.[9]

In other words, the transformation of examples of beneficent and non-maleficent behavior (just like the transformation of examples of autonomous or just behavior) into free-standing principles to be applied to a problematic situation does not improve the human condition, but merely substitutes a "new kind of enslavement,"[10] one that restricts the development of intelligent inquiry, discussion and expression to a pre-determined path. As implied in chapter two, principles ought to be regarded not as restrictions, but as tools, suggested by past conditions and regarded as potential means for addressing current conditions. Obviously, a health care ethics—or an ethical system of any sort—that regards beneficence and non-maleficence solely (or predominantly) as externally-applied principles stipulating certain formal practices and affecting only recipients ignores the realities and seriously underestimates the richness, the vast potentialities and the particular vulnerabilities of our shared, lived experience. Chapter five will examine the cases presented in chapter two from this reconstructed view of beneficence and non-maleficence.

8. JUSTICE AS A BIO/PSYCHO/SOCIAL CONCEPT

There is an ancient Chinese parable that describes heaven and hell as being precisely the same: each is a huge banquet with sumptuous foods placed on round tables. Each person is seated at one of the round tables and given a pair of chopsticks five feet long. In hell, everyone struggles in isolation trying to eat with his own set of chopsticks and eventually starves to death. In heaven, everyone uses his own set of chopsticks to serve the person directly across the table from him and no one goes hungry.

According to the parable, heaven and hell will not be different from the rest of our experiences: they will be what we choose—and/or are led—to make of them. If each person assumes the habit of treating experiences as phenomena that are undergone privately and as the property of an isolated individual self, then developing solutions to problems that are experienced becomes the responsibility of the lone experiencer. On this view, whether individuals seek external consultation with others or not, they are expected and expect themselves to solve "their own" problems. As a consequence, the possibilities that the transformative effects of interdependent and co-operative action can have on both means and ends or goals will remain hidden from view and, thus, undeveloped.

According to conceptions of justice that presuppose persons to be isolated units of self-determination, then, the persons in hell were treated equally and the persons in heaven were treated equally, so both situations are equally just. The effectiveness of the parable lies in its identification of such a conception of equality with hell rather than heaven, because it ignores important bio/psycho/social aspects central to being a person, which includes having a life that is simultaneously characterized by dependence upon and responsibility for others.

On the reconstructed view of persons as bio/psycho/social entities being proposed here, however, the idea of justice is not easily captured by its usual formal expression as the principle that equals are to be treated equally. The view of persons being defended here makes much of the fact that individuals have unique strengths and weaknesses. When entities, because of their particular interrelationships with their environments, have developed unique characteristics, there is an important sense in which simply treating them equally falls short of recognizing and respecting them for what they are.

Nor is the idea of justice more clearly captured by its usual material (as opposed to formal) expression, i.e., that treatment or distribution is to be equal unless morally decisive reasons can be given for unequal treatment or distribution. This cannot occur until the historical context of the social antecedents that determines the bases for distribution is clearly understood and accepted as reasonable and fair. For example, the original intent of public education was to distribute social goods (in this instance, information and knowledgeable teachers) equally. However, when the bulk of funding for each public school site is tied to the revenues generated by the real estate taxes in that particular district, the resulting discrepancy in funding that develops between rich and poor sections of a community is anything but equal. Yet, everyone in the poor districts is treated equally (badly) and everyone in the rich districts is treated equally. In other words, our concept of justice is deeply dependent on the concept of person upon which it is built, and inadequacies in the latter carry over directly as inadequacies in the former.

The Chinese parable captures an important aspect of justice that the conceptions employed in the standard approach ("conceptions" because there are a variety of formulations employed within the approach, all resting on the same set of presuppositions) either miss or consider a peripheral feature: the possibilities of solidarity. On the view being proposed here, seeking justice for oneself entails being sensitive to one's interrelationships with one's environmental field and, especially, to the needs of others. For on this view, it is in the mutually defining features of this fundamental interrelationship that the scope of possible individual freedoms acquires definition and the notion of justice gains concrete substance. However, this can occur only through communication and participation of persons in unhampered, thoughtful and intelligently directed inquiry. The thrust of such an inquiry is to determine what they, as a community of sentient, rational beings with unique perspectives to offer, would collaboratively choose as a reasonable solution to their common problem, given the possibilities available to them due to the constraints of their particular context.

A health care ethics—or a system of ethics of any kind—that regards justice solely as a formal principle, stipulating only what is owed persons by virtue of their status as autonomous individuals, ignores a central fact. It ignores the fact that what counts as justice is neither timeless nor axiomatic. Rather, it is but an attempt to make explicit the implicit norms of our common, and frequently conflicting expectations and actual practices through intelligent inquiry, which includes the social practice of asking and giving reasons. In chapter five, the cases discussed in chapter two will be re-examined from this reconstructed view of justice.

9. CHARACTERIZING THE ETHICAL THROUGH BIO/PSYCHO/SOCIAL CONTEXT

Throughout this work, I have implicitly and explicitly appealed to context as elemental for understanding the origin and nature of ethical obligation between persons. There is nothing novel to this appeal, per se. Certainly, an integral part of modern medical inquiry has always been the individual patient's *story*. Diagnosis requires not only specialized theoretical knowledge and general expertise, but also a specific patient's story. Thus, there is something important that the field of health care has provided the field of ethics: an understanding of the importance of performing, as it were, ethical diagnoses and ethical autopsies. Implicit in such a paradigm is an emphasis in assessing alternative approaches to ethical inquiry that attends better to the particular and concrete in problematic cases by means of stories—negative as well as positive ones.

The patient's story—like *every* story—is the product of an intersubjective process and has an objective status in the sense that it is as real as the patient whose story it is. Included in that story are a history, a physical, a differential diagnosis, a set of possible prognoses (from best case to worst case scenarios) and a range of treatment alternatives. The patient evolves and narrates a *history*. This personal history is corroborated or refuted by family, friends and physical findings. The very fact that such a history can come together about a person and can be communicated and argued about is itself yet another example of the bio/psycho/social context of ethical reflection.

In the health care setting, the health care teams' observations and examinations of and their interactions with the patient generate *physical findings*. These clinicians' assessments of the physical findings and their own specialized knowledge and expertise, in conjunction with the patient's history, generate a *diagnosis* and a *prognosis*. The *range of treatment alternatives* is a joint production of clinicians (based on their expertise) and social institutions (based on their responsibility for deciding which goods and services will be made available for distribution and how they will be distributed). At every point along the way, there is (ideally) a process of collaboration and negotiation between health care team and patient (or her designated representative) that facilitates the resolution of the problematic aspects of the story without closing its consequences off to further re-assessment.

It comes as no great surprise that "telling a story" is so very successful as a method of ethical education and development for persons from childhood on up. For the great stories of our cultural heritages provide descriptions of and commentaries on tacit as well as explicit communal frameworks within which occur the negotiation and development of what come to be considered ethically significant features of experience. They provide a setting within which we can identify, compare, contrast, imaginatively test, evaluate and discuss what have come to be considered ideals, principles, values and virtues within our associations and communities—and to what purpose.

Being confronted with, for example, the Greek tragedies challenges us as individuals to re-examine, set aside, defend or discard any particular point of view (whether personal or cultural) by forcing us to experience the story imaginatively from a multiplicity of often-times competing perspectives. Such stories thereby enrich us in a way that fulfills our need "to see the world whole." They provide us with the opportunity, in a leisurely and safe setting, to pursue alternatives by imaginative rehearsal without actually suffering the consequences. In describing the immense value which great works of literature have for us, Lorraine Code eloquently reminds us:

> Novels may not give us moral knowledge directly and unequivocally, but they often show us ways of placing moral points of view in possible human situations. They illustrate some of the perplexities and implications of putting moral theories into practice so that one can see the importance of certain stances and understanding something of why they will or will not, should or should not work.[11]

The patient/clinician relationship can be aptly viewed as a story that evolves out of multiple perspectives or points of view. Every step of the way in the development of the patient's story there are individuals and disciplines registering and communicating their "take" on circumscribed aspects of the story. This notion of the narrative processing of events—the creative envisioning which occurs within the context of one's knowledge and understanding of one's larger bio/psycho/social possibilities—is, in large part, what makes it possible for persons to understand themselves as beings who have lives.

In addition, attending to the narrative processing of events in any story forces us to recognize that having a point of view is an integral feature of having a life and to realize that others may have points of view that are startlingly different from our own. This is especially true in health care cases, where life and death issues are often so vividly drawn and contested. Taking a perspective different from one's own, seeing how it enhances or diminishes what one claims to value from one's own perspective, is at once humbling and enriching. But, more importantly, it is to engage in behavior that is characteristically ethical. It requires one to engage in representing perspectives other than one's own in the most charitable of terms possible while defending one's own perspective with the most compelling good reasons one can muster. Being able to see an issue from a multiplicity of perspectives is the intellectual tool by which all inquiries (ethical, scientific or otherwise) are progressively refined and advanced; but it is the reflective activity itself, the element of reflective inquiry or intelligence, that is most distinctively called "moral."

According to Martha Nussbaum the real task of moral philosophy is "to make a fine artistic creation" of the "raw" material of experience.[12] This "fine artistic creation" is at once a continuous process and product of persons. It is a bio/psycho/social activity because it is the result of the dynamic interrelations between a certain kind of organism, a person, and its environment. While the "artist" produces her "product" in the first person singular, she is nevertheless an "artist" only by virtue of being a participant in a set of intelligently constructed and directed social practices that occur within a particular physical environment. Between the artist, the artistic community and the wider community there is—both tacitly and explicitly—a continuous intellectual dialogue and narrative that reflects the negotiation involved in the very meaning of what it is to make "a fine artistic creation." So everyone who engages attentively in concrete moral reflection, Nussbaum is saying, is likewise striving to be an artist in this sense.

Medicine is also an art—but it is an art predicated on the sciences. In our culture, a dichotomy between art and science is widely accepted; but as chapter three explained, Dewey rejected such deep dichotomies between the varieties of reflective inquiry. Science, perceptively understood, is the result of the dynamic interrelations between a certain kind of organism and its environment, it is bio/psycho/social through and through. This is the reason, this one not yet well examined, that the scientific and artistic elements of medical practice are not at constant war, because their deepest roots are recognized to be one and the same. And this is also why ethical inquiry need not be at war with the scientific side of health care practice.

Good outcomes in health care cannot be reduced to physiological statistics simply by virtue of the fact that treating patients presupposes quantitative laboratory data; but a proper bio/psycho/social understanding of science offers no basis for such a reductive conclusion in the first place.

Reflecting about ethical issues in health care encounters requires understanding physics, chemistry, pathophysiology, psychology and sociology; but this does not mean that ethics or philosophical reflection about it can be exhausted by, reduced to or passively read off of these sciences.

Ethical reflection within the health care setting calls upon scientists at work there to remember the bio/psycho/social grounds of their forms of reflective inquiry. In a parallel way, ethical analysis in the field of health care calls upon the fields of ethics and philosophy to remember that reflective inquiry—the *sine qua non* of ethics and philosophy—because it is a characteristic of persons, is a never-ending piecemeal project that represents the activity of a particular sort of organism's dynamic interreation with its environment.

An approach to ethics which ignores these considerations is one which, in the real world, lacks flexibility and leads to premature closure. It is premature, not in the sense that all data necessary to a particular case's disposition have not been gathered and sufficiently scrutinized. Rather, it is premature in the sense that the totality of the whole problem as it extends into the future can no longer be viewed dynamically. In other words, a "solution" can become reified and made to serve as a fixed solution to future problems rather than as a springboard to further exploration of a complex and dynamic issue. When this occurs, principles such as autonomy, beneficence, non-maleficence and justice are treated as isolated set pieces to be externally applied to problems rather than as elements of on-going reflection already part of an indeterminate situation.

Adopting a bio/psycho/social view of ethical reflection requires us to look at persons and their problems as part and parcel of a more extensive project. This project aims not at closure but at seeking to bring about a pragmatic "end-in-view"—i.e., a temporary end that serves to deal with an immediate problem—as a means towards further reflective inquiry, learning and intellectual growth for the future. In such a view of ethical reflection, resolutions are means to further inquiry that will be made necessary by the dynamic bio/psycho/social network or field in which persons are embedded. That is, the persons, the data (of which principles and all the fruits of previous ethical reflection are but a part) and the environmental context (of which each community as it is at any given moment is a part) in which such problem solving occurs are dynamically interactive. Even though the resolutions may, across cases at different times, be the same, problems are still not to be considered merely as challenges met, once and for all.

The approach offered here looks at each problem and its resolution as always at once both an ad hoc resolution of an indeterminacy and an indication of a larger challenge in progress which can only be "met" in the same way: progressively. Such an approach is far more flexible and adaptive to the needs of persons as we actually find them because it allows for change, is open to the new data that the reflective life reveals and, therefore, actively seeks to re-examine prior decisions in the light of changing circumstance.

However, describing the approach without solidifying *it* into an algorithm is challenging. Before saying any more about it—both for clarity's sake and because this is what the approach itself requires—the three cases examined in chapter two will now be re-examined.

ENDNOTES

1. John Dewey, *LW* 2:299.
2. These Greek concepts were used similarly by Thomasine Kushner in an attempt to bring some clarity to the abortion issue in an article entitled "Having a Life versus Being Alive," *Journal of Medical Ethics*, 1984, 1: 5-8.
3. Evidence of the confusion of these two concepts in the English language can be seen by our appropriation of "bios" in the word, biology, instead of the more appropriate connection this field of study has to "zoe."
4. The section entitled "Dewey's Pragmatic Theory of Experience" in chapter three contains several quotes from Dewey's description of the organism/environment interrelationship that makes individuation possible.
5. Dewey, *LW* 12:32.
6. The concept of "basic need" is a complex issue in its own right, and it is beyond the scope of this work to give it the space and time that it would require. Therefore, for the purposes of this work, I will simply use Erich H. Loewy's distinction of basic needs as either "first-order necessities," (i.e., those means requisite for sustaining the immediate goals of biological existence—air, nourishment and shelter being prime examples) or "second-order basic necessities," (i.e., those means required to sustain existence within a given social context so that an individual can effectively pursue having a life—health care and education being prime examples). See Erich H. Loewy, *Textbook of Healthcare Ethics*, 2nd ed. (New York: Plenum Press, 1996), pp. 245-48.
7. Dewey, *LW* 2:352-3.
8. The term, "mentor," originated in Greek mythology. Mentor, a wise teacher, was asked by his close friend, Odysseus, to watch over his young son, Telemachus. Mentor acted as a surrogate parent, supporting and protecting Telemachus while gently guiding and nurturing him towards adulthood. In Homer's *Odyssey*, Telemachus is accompanied in his search for his father, Odysseus, by Athene, the goddess of wisdom, who disguises herself as Mentor, knowing that the mutual bond forged between Telemachus and Mentor will, in the process, secure Telemachus' trust and provide the participatory setting necessary for acquiring wisdom.
9. Dewey, *LW* 11:25.
10. Idem.
11. Lorraine Code, *Epistemic Responsibility*, (Hanover, NH: University Press of New England, 1987), p. 225.
12. Martha Nussbaum, "'Finely Aware and Richly Responsible': Moral Attention and the Moral Task of Literature," *Journal of Philosophy*, (1985, 516-29), p. 528.

Chapter 5

Re-assessing the Cases Presented in Chapter Two from a Bio/psycho/social Perspective

1. INTRODUCTION

The goal of this final chapter is to show how the particular approach and reconstructed view of personhood espoused in this work, captures some of the more troubling aspects and problematic features of the cases that the standard approach either misses or is ill prepared to address. This approach differs in several respects from the one used to represent the standard approach in chapter two. While this alternative, too, emphasizes the importance of investigating the respective biological, psychological and social aspects of cases, it's method of investigation differs significantly from that of the standard approach.

One important difference is that the alternative offered here rejects as misguided and/or fruitless the need to find some entirely neutral, generic and disinterested perspective. Misguided because persons are *not* identical, programmable machines but unique individuals with differing backgrounds, goals, desires, needs and interests—indeed, it is precisely this unique individuality that gives ethical problems their characteristic complexity and ambiguity. Fruitless because, given this fact of individuality, there would always be the problem of determining *whose* interpretation of a "neutral, generic and disinterested perspective" ought to take precedence. The alternative approach offered here attempts to accommodate and to represent as many perspectives of the relationship as possible. This includes perspectives with regard to time (i.e., past, present and future) as well as to place (i.e., charitable, yet, fair representations of the perspectives of each of those individuals relevantly affected by the case, its possible resolutions and their consequences).

Another important difference is that the alternative approach denies that "problem-solving" is predominantly a process of discovery and application. In other words, it denies that the purpose of discovery is to yield some *a priori* (pre-existing) solution that preserves the right, the good and the true. And it denies that such a discovery can then be applied to "solve" problems. It also denies that problem-solving can be construed as the solitary pursuit of an observer insulated from the effects of her choices. Instead, it replaces the traditional notion of "problem-solving" as the *end* of inquiry with the much richer notion of "resolution," which emphasizes the transitional nature of the enterprise.

"Resolution" is thus characterized as a collaborative effort, a process that demands creativity and foresight as well as discovery. It is *not* simply the discovery of the one and only "Right, Good and True" solution for all time. Rather, it is a discovery of empirical facts about the existence of an array of competing goods, rights and truths that everything in our experience confirms. It is a process that spans past, present and future insofar as it requires us—in light of our present experience of existence and the distilled wisdom of others' past experiences—to sort out the various competing rights, goods and truths in each particular case. Thus, *together* we may craft a resolution that is, all things considered (and, until the monitoring of it's consequences tell us otherwise), the least wrong, the least bad, the least false.

For, as already remarked in the concluding paragraphs of chapter two, ethics is not about choosing between right and wrong, good and bad, truth or falsity; nor is it a private determination from some neutral, disinterested and insulated vantage point. Rather, ethics is concerned with the much more interesting and collaborative work of attempting to craft a resolution that will affect—whether subtly or dramatically—the life and personality of everyone involved, a resolution that even those most negatively affected will be able to accept. Thus, much of the work of resolution in the alternative approach depends upon the careful sorting out of a whole set of ancillary problems associated with how to proceed in the face of the indeterminate features and ambiguities of each particular case. That is, this approach borrows the Socratic strategy of public, participatory discourse (without the metaphysical baggage of Platonic essentialism) described in chapter one. It has all of those relevantly affected (or their legitimate representatives) involved in the case working collaboratively in asking and answering the three questions: "Where have you come from?" "Where are you going?" "How do we get there?"

As a result, the process (both the asking and the answering) is *personal* insofar as it is performed by, and affects, those individuals party to the relationship. But, just as importantly, the process is also *public* insofar as it is accessible to—and, thus, subject to challenge by—all involved in or relevantly affected by the relationship. Somewhat similar to the manner in which Thomasma and Pellegrino make explicit the plurality of "goods" involved in health care encounters,[1] this alternative approach attempts to render intelligible the even wider plurality of inexplicit, and oftentimes conflicting, interconnected features and interests largely responsible for the existence of such a plurality of "goods."

This is a crucial part of the approach since, it is only insofar as our hidden, half-formed and, as yet, uncritically entertained intuitions about what is of value to us (interests, intentions, means and ends or goals, etc.) are explicitly confronted and subjected to critical, public scrutiny. For it is only then that their coherence, consistency and reasonableness (or lack thereof) become evident to us. In other words, the process itself—as well as its potential means and ends or goals—is bio/psycho/social through and through. Thus, if we are to fully appreciate and make effective use of the fact of our bio/psycho/social existence, this process is not simply *open* to collaborative inquiry; it *requires* it.

At this juncture, several things need to be stressed. First, the fact that it is impossible for all parties to an encounter to discover everything about each other's history does not mean that the attempt to do so is either misguided or futile. Persons cannot recognise, assess or appreciate each other's strengths, weaknesses, wants and needs simply by privately assuming things about one another. Direct and explicit communication between persons, even though it may be fallible or incomplete, is still the surest way to prevent or correct misguided subjective assumptions, as well intentioned as they might be. Second, critics of this alternative approach may complain that, in the real world, no one has time to make explicit all of the myriad assumptions they have to make in order to get on with their daily lives. But if what is desired by persons is to *have* lives (*bios*, not merely *zoe*)—and to make life less indeterminate—then a critical part of accomplishing these things requires more. It requires the kind of explicit, honest, open, charitable and wholehearted intercommunication that characterizes reflective inquiry and participatory discourse as espoused by this alternative approach.

The first question, "Where have you come from?" describes the biographical lives of the persons actively involved in a case. This bio/psycho/social history needs to be asked and answered as early as possible in the health care relationship—ideally, *before* problematic situations become crises. This question is crucial insofar as it allows the participants to assess the collaborative potential of the relationship, thereby allowing more time, if need be, to arrange for an alternative relationship that may better fit the expectations of those most intimately affected.

Moreover, since the biographies of those involved in the health care relationship do continue to evolve, the need to re-ask this first question can always arise. However, because it ordinarily describes individual sets of fairly established personal habits and interests (at least in adults), the presumption is that the initial answers to this first question should not be subject to abrupt changes without reasons that can be articulated and understood even when those reasons or their implications may be controversial.

The second question, "Where are you going?" while shaped by history and present circumstance, anticipates the viability and future possibilities of the relationship by elucidating the goals, values and expectations of each of the participants to the relationship in light of the physical and technical limitations of the situation. In the event that any of the participants' goals, values or expectations cannot be reconciled by consensus or reasonable compromise, the second question illuminates the limitations—perhaps even the non-viability—of the relationship as heretofore conceived and the need for seeking an alternative.

Moreover, as the membership of the relationship may change and the bio/psycho/social (including medical) situation of the patient and the other personae will evolve over the course of time, so the answer to this second question may also change over time. Therefore, this question needs frequent re-asking and re-answering, especially whenever the patient's medical condition changes, but also simply whenever any of the participants to the relationship have reason to believe that a re-assessment is warranted.

The third question, "How do we get there?" presupposes that a great deal of the necessary consensus and compromise entailed by the constraints of the first two questions has already been accomplished. However, there is still much information to learn, share, discuss and re-assess on a continuing basis. So, how the third question is asked and answered will be prompted by and may, in turn, prompt re-assessment of the other two questions.

This third question, because it deals predominantly with means, presupposes the explicit as well as tacit involvement of the larger community in ways that the first two questions may not, since the technology often required is largely created, controlled and allocated by the social institutions of the community. This serves as a reminder of the depth and intricacy of the bio/psycho/social interconnectedness of what in the past has been regarded as, and still is too often considered to be, a simple, dyadic patient/health care clinician relationship. Even in the "good old days," this was an idealization rarely, if ever, actualized. As suggested in chapter one and argued from a Deweyan perspective in chapter three, a central characteristic of the process of intelligent inquiry, whether the subject matter is viewed as science or morals, is openness to the challenge of re-asking, re-entertaining and re-answering these three questions at any point along the way.

Before returning to the three cases analysed in chapter two, some further cautionary remarks are in order. First, to reduce overlap and undue repetition, those aspects of a case that remain unchanged from the first analysis to the second will simply be assumed without explicit repetition. Those aspects that are substantially changed, however, will be clearly noted and their circumstances carefully established and addressed.

Second, because we are not actually participants in these cases and do not actually enter into them as they progress in real time—i.e., we are only thinking them through and not *also* undergoing them—these analyses cannot go beyond the level of imaginative rehearsal. That is, a central aspect of the reconstruction of these cases will be missing: namely, the evolutionary modifications that develop in the course of the normal give and take of actual participation in a case resolution. However, given the empiricist constraints of the method of science, this should not be considered a defect of the enterprise, but one of its characteristic features. Until these prospective modifications actually occur and the breadth and depth of *all* of their effects can be measured, assessed, compared with customary practice and reviewed, there can be no hard evidence for or against their efficacy. (The reader would be well-advised to re-read that last sentence several times, remembering that, until how modifications actually do affect both the agent (and her future actions) and the entire environment she is acting upon are factored in as well, evaluation will, in crucial ways, remain incomplete.)

Given the track record of the experimental sciences as examples of successful models of reflective inquiry, and so of this approach, one can reasonably anticipate that, whatever prospective and preventive strategies are used to resolve cases such as those examined here, if they are to be consistent with a bio/psycho/social approach, will eventually have to include critical scrutiny and revision of those social institutions associated with health care. This should make them more accessible and responsive to the persons they serve.

For the convenience of the reader, each of the following re-analyses will be prefaced by the case as it was originally presented in chapter two.

2. CASE ANALYSES

2.1 Case 1: The "Rescue Medicine" Conundrum

During a recent cold winter an indigent, elderly man was brought into a local emergency room with pneumonia. He was close to starvation and suffered from hypothermia because he could not afford to eat or heat his room after paying his rent. While in the emergency room, the man suffered a cardiac arrest. Three weeks after aggressive cardio-pulmonary resuscitation and stabilization, he remained completely unresponsive and totally dependent on a ventilator. During this time social services discovered that the man had no family or friends. The health care team suspected that the patient would remain permanently comatose, and a neurological consult confirmed the team's suspicion that the patient's prognosis was bleak.

An ethicist was consulted to discuss whether it was ethically appropriate to discontinue this man's treatment and was told by the health care team that between $100,000 and $200,000 had been expended treating this man. The members of the health care team concurred that, had it been possible to restore the patient to a semblance of his pre-hospitalization condition (which it was not), they would have felt no qualms about continuing treatment. Such treatment would have, in effect, returned this patient to the material conditions responsible for his hospitalization in the first place.

2.1.1 Analysis

The analysis of this case in chapter two ended with the health care team having decided to withdraw all of this patient's medical treatment with the exception of comfort measures. The reasoning behind this decision was based on the assumption that this patient would not wish to be sustained in a vegetative existence. This assumption, in turn, was based on the belief that most persons having the opportunity to decide this issue in advance would not choose to be sustained in a vegetative state. (Might this explain the perennial concern in the literature about providing comfort measures for patients who are in a vegetative existence?) On the basis of these assumptions it was argued that the principles of autonomy, beneficence, non-maleficence and justice would best be served, and the values they represent best maximized by withdrawing all treatment except comfort measures.

The account of individualism that is assumed in this reasoning and implied in the standard approach, includes the presupposition that respecting a person entails treating her—or, in this instance, him—as an isolated, insulated locus of rational self-determination and self-sufficiency. The rationale behind this account appears to be as follows: because certain characteristics are worthy of respect (e.g., rationality, self-determination, self-sufficiency), the class of entities having those characteristics are, in turn, worthy of respect. However, reliance on this account of individualism to justify treatment decisions for patients in circumstances like those of this case is not defensible since it is precisely these characteristics (along with others) of personhood that are missing or seriously compromised in this patient. Hence, this account of individualism cannot adequately make sense of the notion of ethical obligations in such a case.

For an account of individualism to be considered adequate, it must take seriously the antecedent experiential context and conditions of personhood. That is, it must attend to the fact that a person's distinctive features—those characteristics that make her who she is—are not the product of a lone, disinterested and completely self-sufficient author. Rather, they are the result of a continuous and dynamic bio/psycho/social process, an active, dynamic expression of that particular individual's interdependent relationships with her environment. The alternative approach advocated here espouses this richer, reconstructed account of individualism and its implications. Among other things, it enables us to make sense of why we still feel the tug of ethical obligation to persons whose autonomy has been seriously compromised. In short, it grounds the notion of ethical obligation *not* in some independent, neutral criteria that define what it is to be a person, but in the particular bio/psycho/social matrix of that individual's existence as a person.

In other words, when an individual, such as the patient in this case, permanently loses those characteristics that make it possible for him to *have* a life, the ethical alternatives of those others connected with his situation are not limited simply to speculating about what some generic person would want when he is no longer capable of appreciating his situation or making that choice. Rather, in the event that a patient cannot directly act or speak for himself, every attempt is made to reconstruct his particular perspective and then to represent it with as much accuracy and fidelity as possible.

That is why the ethical obligations of those involved in caring for such a patient cannot be determined from applying a set of independently derived principles. On the contrary, every attempt must be made to reconstruct that particular patient's story—his bio/psycho/social history, his unique relationship with his environment. This alternative account of personhood, because it is committed to attempting such a reconstruction of the person's perspective, makes it possible to talk coherently about ethical obligations to patients who, according to the standard approach's account of individualism, are no longer rational, self-determined or self-sufficient.

Taking the bio/psycho/social matrix of ethical obligation seriously also reinforces a particular kind of collaborative process that distinguishes this alternative approach from the standard approach in a very important respect; namely, it is a *homeostatic* collaborative process. That is to say, this process is not simply causal, nor simply reactive. Rather, it is *homeostatic*, insofar as the dynamic balance sought in this particular kind of collaboration is one that promotes the integrity of the whole by protecting the integrity of each of the individual elements involved, and this includes the interrelationships that characterize those individual elements.

This homeostatic collaboration is guided by the Deweyan notion of "intelligence." As such, it meets those requirements of reflective inquiry that were discussed earlier in chapter three: (1) active engagement, (2) publicity, (3) effort towards the mutual understanding of and respect for differences, (4) openness to the inevitability of modification or change and (5) willingness to allow ourselves to be led by the dynamic of the inquiry rather than by pre-established interests and expectations (whether they be private or public). This notion of intelligence is quite different from a process in which pre-established principles are applied (however intelligently) algorithmically, analogous to the way in which men are deployed against one another in a game of chess, until one side or the other is victorious.

If this alternative account of individualism were incorporated into ethical analyses of health care encounters, a corresponding change in the scope, structure and function of professional codes and formal statements about the primary goals and values of health care would also follow. The general focus of these formal ideals of health care practice would still be to benefit individual patients. However, because "patient" and "benefit" would be more broadly construed, from within a bio/psycho/social perspective, both theory and practice in health care would be significantly altered.

In other words, because it enhances our understanding of how profoundly the antecedent conditions (especially the social ones) of our current environment influence what it is to be a *person*—that is, not merely to *be* alive but to *have* a life—this alternative account would (1) enable finer distinctions to be drawn at the level of each particular case, (2) make it easier to translate formal statements into effective guides to action and (3) prompt the creation, interaction and evolution of the kinds of flexible social structures that can anticipate as well as respond to cases such as this one. As a result, our social institutions will be better equipped to deal with such cases prospectively—viz., before a person ends up unconscious, at the door of an emergency room somewhere.

Compare, for example, the items (listed on page 23) that are traditionally included in formal statements about the primary goals and values of the health care professions with the following list which, due to the broader perspective suggested by this alternative approach, represents a difference in emphasis as well as scope:

1. Promoting health through education
2. Relieving symptoms, pain and, when possible, suffering
3. Maintaining and improving function or minimizing its deterioration
4. Avoiding exposure of patients to gratuitous harm or unnecessary risk

5. Curing (as opposed to merely prolonging biological life) whenever possible
6. Providing comfort measures and/or orchestrating death when curing or maintaining functional life (i.e., bios) is precluded

Obviously, these items, like those originally listed on page 23, may differ in emphasis or ranking, depending upon the particular case at issue. However, it should be noticed that, in making explicit the differences in the antecedent and consequent elements between *having* a life and *being* alive, the alternative bio/psycho/social approach changes the focus of these primary goals and values. It changes it from one that is merely static and reactionary to one that is dynamic, critical and prospective.

As a result, rather than being required to respond to a series of events that they had no hand in creating, the persons involved are in a better position to guide rather than only be guided by events. Instead of re-affirming the presumption that the primary role of clinicians and patients alike requires them to react individually to aspects of an encounter as though responding to a series of isolated and immediate "givens," this alternative approach requires the accommodation and collaboration of both patients and clinicians in anticipating, understanding and resolving problematic elements of an encounter. And, at times, it may require accommodation and collaboration beyond the immediate confines of any one particular encounter. When, for example, clinicians begin to find that their encounters with patients share certain problematic elements with increasing frequency (say, for example, the managed care facility in which they work has a policy that systematically interferes with certain expensive, but medically indicated treatments), a habit of professional collaborative discourse and resolution would make it far less likely for individual clinicians to feel isolated and overwhelmed by the issue. As a result, it would lower the threshold for collective action of the part of clinicians, paving the way for an earlier and more effective response to the issue. In other words, the alternative, bio/psycho/social approach considered here makes it possible for *all* of the persons involved (clinicians as well as patients) to *have* lives—to become (or remain) subjects of their lives—in ways that simply cannot be accomplished by (putative) lone individuals.

However, replacing a principlist applications model of problem-solving like the standard approach with a prospective and participatory one, and moving therefore beyond a crisis management mode of intervention to one that emphasizes prevention entails change. It entails the development of a different set of practices between persons and a different set of commitments and expectations between persons and their social institutions than currently exists. Hence, even more so than in the other two cases still to be reanalysed, this particular case illustrates how the alternative approach would reconstruct the way health care-related social institutions currently function, in order to prevent—or, at least, to minimize—the occurrence of such cases. To see the practical implications of this claim more clearly, it is helpful to understand the limitations of current health care practice.

In current practice it is a commonplace that, once a person gains access to health care services, the standard of that care is unaffected by what are considered extraneous, i.e., non-medical, considerations, and resources are frequently treated as if they were infinite. The delivery system of our health care institution has developed in such a way as to insulate clinicians from patients in several important ways. First, it insulates clinicians from persons and their lives until they present either with discrete medical complaints or, less frequently, with specific concerns for preventing illness and/or learning how to develop healthier lifestyles. Second, it insulates clinicians from those aspects of their patients' lives that are not considered relevant either to the diagnosis and treatment of the immediate pathophysiology or pathopsychology that prompted the patient to seek medical care or to the patient's specific concerns with prevention and self-care.

This insulation has unwittingly led to a number of difficulties, the most notable being the change wrought in the clinicians' focus of concern. It has increasingly been diverted from patients as persons having lives to patients as isolated sets of symptoms. And it has been diverted from the on-going challenge of educating and engaging persons in their own preventive and maintenance care (since even preventive care today is usually in response to a quite circumscribed crisis or feared crisis). Instead, the focus of concern shifts to the time-slice drama of rescue medicine, with its emphasis on crisis management and need for technology that is labor-intensive and, more likely than not, quite expensive.

As a result, clinicians currently expend huge amounts of time, effort and resources rescuing individuals from medical problems that often are unwittingly induced or exacerbated by existing social arrangements, arrangements that may have been instituted to prevent or ameliorate some other existing social problem. In other words, many of the medical problems that clinicians must deal with today exist as a consequence of attempts to address causative factors of social and psycho/social conditions as though they were themselves independent of and, thus, incapable of affecting health and health care.

As exemplified in this case, involvement of clinicians too often is limited to a person's hospitalization for a very discrete, but artificially isolated problem. The clinicians in this case have been insulated very effectively not only from the social roots of this person's condition. They have also been insulated for the most part, from the kind of prospective collaboration with other social organizations and institutions that could prevent or minimize the occurrence of just such cases as his.

Another major source of difficulty is the way that the standard approach interprets clinicians' obligations in relation to health care resources. A commitment to fulfill the goals of health care professionals, as these are conventionally understood within the standard approach, presupposes unlimited access to the resources necessary to provide that care. The fact of the matter, of course, is that health care resources have always been limited and, as our society is just beginning to realize, it simply could not be otherwise. Therefore, that these professionals experience ethical conflict is inevitable. The goals and guiding principles of health care clinicians are inconsistent with the economic goals and intentions of the larger community. Yet, there is nothing in the standard approach to assist health care professionals in resolving this conflict because its focus in practice is always limited to the patient/clinician relationship, and not that relationship's larger psycho/social context.

As our society now faces ever-increasing budgetary difficulties, resources are being treated less cavalierly in the larger society and health care is therefore becoming even more difficult to deliver. Clinicians are also being asked to help conserve resources. They are being told that for too long they have been insulated from the "real" world, the world of limited access and limited resources. But to expect clinicians to act in the face of these conflicting demands, each demand supported by arguments from the same narrow set of principles, without at the same time actively reconstructing the approach to ethical reflection that is being undertaken, is to invite them to compromise their professional commitments. It asks them to subordinate the needs of individual patients to the economic interests *of certain segments* of their society.

The introduction of the concept and practice of "managed care," for example, has only served to heighten this conflict by placing clinicians, especially physicians, in the position of weighing the health care needs of their patients directly against their own economic well-being. It is always interesting, by the way, to listen what most people *mean* when they speak about resources. Invariably, they mean *material* resources. Oh, we pay lip-service to non-material resources—such as expertise, time, effort, personal commitment, loyalty, trustworthiness—but few of us are prepared to discuss, let alone attempt to factor into the resource equation, the benefits and burdens of continuing to ignore the importance of non-material resources.

Unlike the alternative approach espoused here, the prevalent view of the responsibility of clinicians to patients, like the standard approach which grounds it, is not understood to include health care professionals undertaking a prospective critique of the means and ends or goals of existing social institutions. Nor is this responsibility thought to include providing services that other social institutions have failed to cover. Echoing a long-standing view of human relationships in our society, the health care professions' attitudes have overwhelmingly been that their members' professional obligations are limited to the symptomatic treatment of individual, identified patients having specific, circumscribed complaints.

Notice in this connection, for example, the language standardly used to record a patient's complaint upon hospital admission: "This patient presents with..." The health care team is "presented" with an already circumscribed and isolated problem. While a patient's history and physical is done to try to establish the reasons for the troubling situation, routinely formulating the problem in this way biases the inquiry. That is, clinicians are expected to identify and to focus on correcting only those physiological antecedents directly responsible for an isolated phenomenon and/or on counseling the patient to modify personal habits contributing directly to it. Therefore, their efforts are antecedently structured to deal with these cases in isolation from their contexts instead of, for example, helping the public to recognize and to come to terms with the larger, more extensive social roots of the ills these cases reveal.

This is why such problematic cases currently tend to be discussed as though they were isolated phenomena to be resolved—and the resolution justified—retrospectively and within a tightly circumscribed context. The antecedent conditions and potential consequences of a case are considered relevant only as they directly concern the patient at hand in his or her current condition or those other persons (e.g., family members) actively and directly involved in the case as it is presently being addressed. As a result, the deeper, underlying social antecedents and consequents of an issue are never addressed because they are not even recognized as part of the problem.

Unless compelling reasons can be given to show that the bio/psycho/social conditions of personhood, of *having* a life, can safely be ignored, the ethical obligations of the health care team must be reconstructed. Such obligations must extend beyond purely biological and technical considerations to include the psycho/social. In other words, the presuppositions of the standard approach need to be reconstructed to view health care as a socially situated response of socially situated individuals. It must be understood as an element of a continually problematic human world—but also one that, because fallible, is, fortunately for us all, always potentially correctable. Once that reconstruction is properly undertaken, the nature of ethical obligation—that it is a situated response bound up in the co-operative interrelationships and collaborative practices of having a life—will become clearer. Such corrections could then be anticipated and instituted—if not before the oftentimes subtle, but far-reaching burdensomeness of certain practices was felt, then at least earlier rather than later along the way.

Though widely prevalent, the view of health care being criticized here is not universal. Many clinicians here in our country do recognize that this sort of isolation and insulation is a falsification of the real world. They understand that fully addressing this patient's situation in this case would require taking into account the social environment this man comes from and its causal role in his medical condition, as well as his understanding of the health care system and his comprehension of his situation, etc. They understand that their commitment to patients requires concern for the environment people live in and see the connection between their profession and social and political action.

That is, even though such concerns are considered additional and optional under the current view of the obligations of health care professionals here in the United States, there are, both recently and historically, important exceptions. Clinicians, and physicians especially, have found themselves at the forefront of social action. They have functioned as activists lobbying for social change, from nineteenth century public health reforms[2] to organizing against nuclear war in this century.[3] The most recent group of activist physicians—*Médecin sans frontiéres*, translated into English as "Doctors without Borders"—is French-based, but includes physicians from all over the world, including the United States. The organization is dedicated to providing temporary medical assistance in times of natural disasters, wars and political or social upheavals.

What these individuals and groups have in common is a recognition that social and political decisions apparently remote from health care can place whole groups of persons at risk medically. They have held and currently hold that health care professionals have a vital role in addressing the underlying problematic sources of these issues, not simply patient-by-patient, but globally—i.e., socially—because of their status as experts in health care and the special obligations that status confers. Accordingly, there is precedent for the claim that clinicians should understand that their commitment to individual, identified patients requires concern for and responsiveness to the social and political conditions under which individuals become patients. But, advocates of the standard approach and of the conventional understanding of obligations of health care professions have addressed this position almost not at all, much less provided health care clinicians with active guidance about how it might be carried out.

So, it is not surprising that the clinicians involved in the first case were troubled. It is likely that this patient was already in the process of becoming socially abandoned long before his present medical needs were significant and that the medical treatment he required when he "presented" was probably a direct result of that abandonment. This is deeply and cruelly ironic since, just in monetary terms alone, the amount spent for his hospitalization on this one occasion could have kept him—and a number of others in similar straits—in rent, food and adequate heat for well over the entire winter. But the current practices of the larger social system (and the presuppositions that support them) not only permit, but also actively underwrite, his abandonment. The standard approach encourages us to regard his medical needs and their treatment as discrete facts rather than integrally connected aspects of human life in a social world. The assumptions about persons and their lives presumed by the standard approach work to shape professional ethical thinking in precisely this way.

To re-iterate, then: the belief that the material conditions of this man's existence outside of the contingent circumstances of his hospitalization have no bearing on the health care team's ethical obligations to patients precisely misses the point of who this patient is and why he is where he is. To understand this point is to challenge the conception of the clinician/patient relationship as isolated person (or team of persons)-to-isolated person (or person plus significant others). It is to require, in its place, one that conceives of each pole of this relationship as being situated much more richly and meaningfully—and, therefore, ambiguously—within a broad social context, a context that eventually includes, among other things, the entire institutional and societal distribution system.

While some conflict is inevitable in any society, it is certainly not unrealistic to expect that social institutions and their access (especially in a democracy) be restructured when they no longer serve as effective means for empowering individuals in ways that also benefit and strengthen the community as a whole. However, this cannot occur so long as these institutions are regarded merely as providers of isolated services or products. In reality, social agencies and institutions, at their best, "provide" only one thing: a communicative forum, an intellectual space within which individuals can come together to arrange ways in which they can prospectively share their strengths and thereby minimize the effects of their weaknesses. This means that, if problems in health care are to be adequately addressed, the opinions and advice of all sorts of experts—in health care, philosophy, history, economics, psychology, cultural anthropology, sociology, etc.—must be prospectively sought. This expert advice must be disseminated to the public who, only then, can intelligently participate in the discussion and debate necessary to critique and to improve and/or replace existing strategies for resolving these problems.

Of course, individual health care providers might rightly fear in this matter what could be called the "slippery-slope of obligation." It is a fear that, once involved in the resolution of psycho/social aspects of specific cases, the floodgates will be opened and there will be no end to their responsibility for people. Very possibly clinicians would then be diverted from effecting diagnosis, prognosis and treatment—matters about which they have been trained—and they would become responsible for a host of psycho/social interventions that they are unskilled in performing and for which they have been given no effective institutional supports. In truth, given the current structure of our social institutions and the prevailing view of the responsibilities of clinicians to patients, these fears are probably justified. In this country today, clinicians are trained—and rewarded—for short-term, circumscribed and technically sophisticated medical rescue. If the public's expectations about the range of rescue interventions increases without an accompanying reconstruction and clarification of clinicians' obligations (and possibly preparation) vis à vis society's obligations (in this instance, to provide appropriate, equitable, efficient and timely resource allocation, etc.), then our society's health care professionals will be caught in an even worse bind than the bio/psycho/socially sensitive among them presently face.

There is no straightforward way in this country's present health care system for clinicians to counsel society to modify its habits, institutions and ways of ethical thinking about patients and health care. In fact, the focus of most of our public health programs has been almost exclusively to protect society from the spread of disease by isolating the ill (e.g., victims of plague), establishing and monitoring sanitation codes and overseeing inoculation programs.[4] In other words, what are even recognized as legitimate social health care goals and appropriate possible courses of action are similarly determined by the presuppositions about persons, relationships and obligation on which they rest. So, the analysis and application of underlying intuitions—even the reconstructed ones tentatively set out in chapter four—serve no effective purpose unless and until persons come together to devise methods for identifying the underlying sources of problems (especially when those sources that are political or social) and co-ordinating the effective use of our social resources and institutions towards their resolution. In the remaining sections of this chapter, I will suggest several possible remedies to this current, widespread lack.

2.2 Case 2: Medical Treatment For A Social Ill

> A frail, elderly man without relatives or visitors has lived in an extended care facility for the past five years. While needing physical assistance with daily activities, such as bathing and walking, he is oriented to time and place. With increasing frequency over the past two years the following pattern of behavior is observed: the patient abruptly informs his health care providers that he will no longer take fluids or food because he wants to die.

Within several days, the man becomes semi-comatose and is sent to the nearest emergency room where he is re-hydrated by means of intravenous fluids and/or naso-gastric intubation. Upon recovery, he consistently expresses regret that he is still alive and disappointment with his caretakers for having over-ridden his wishes. The patient temporarily resumes adequate consumption of fluids and food, only to repeat the cycle in a few months' time.

2.2.1 Analysis

The analysis of this case in chapter two ended with the health care team in the unenviable position of being forced to choose between what they considered to be "the lesser of two evils:" allowing this man to choose death or "forcing" him to live. Namely, they felt forced to choose the option of continuing to send this patient, when he becomes medically unstable and semi-comatose, to the emergency room to be medically treated for his self-induced dehydration and starvation and, in the interim, attempting to dissuade him from persisting in his pattern of behavior. The rationale behind this decision was derived from an understanding of the criteria for decisional capacity based on the atomistic view of individualism espoused by the standard approach. According to this perspective, the principles of autonomy, beneficence and justice would best be served by respecting the patient's rationality and self-determination until he becomes semi-comatose. At that point, the primary injunction, "do no harm," would take precedence and the caregivers would be bound by their professions' general "default" assumptions about the principle of non-maleficence.

Frankly, there is something almost too tidy about this solution. Why should clinicians, once this patient lacks both the freedom to act and the freedom to articulate his will, feel "ethically justified" in carrying out an action that, only a short time before, was considered taboo because it was clearly against this patient's will as he had consistently articulated it? Is it because we really think that the patient might now, after such consistent prior behavior, suddenly relent and, because we now have no way of knowing this, we must always "err on the side of life?" (But doesn't the very language, "err on the side of life,"—an honest sentiment not infrequently voiced by clinicians—beg the question in this particular case?) Or is it more likely because we failed to see the whole fabric of this man's existence as the person he is? Unfortunately, this type of response is not rare, especially in an atmosphere where clinicians, struggling to find ways to protect the integrity of their practices, are pressed to treat symptoms and episodes rather than whole patients.

Certainly, nothing in this man's life situation had changed sufficiently to give us reason to suspect that he would want to abandon the way he'd already decided the rest of his life should go. Yet, it is almost as though the clinicians were confronted, in one time-slice, by a patient with decisional capacity, asserting and pursuing his reflectively thought out choices, and in the next time-slice, by a patient without these capacities, over whom they are not only justified, but required, to assert an entirely ahistorical substituted judgment! In this manner of thinking, the patient in the first time-slice has no necessary connection with the patient in the second time-slice. But why should this man's semi-comatose state suddenly render him a generic ahistorical persona and require us to invoke the old maxim, "Err on the side of life?"

Such a maxim is of undoubted use in cases where we are dealing with a completely unknown patient or questionable situation. It is quite useful in cases where we need to preserve the means—zoe (being alive)—until we can ascertain whether there is, in fact, an end or goal—bios (having a life)—to preserve. But to do so in situations akin to this man's, where we already have a fairly clear understanding of what would constitute acceptable ends or goals for such patients is, to say the least, peculiarly inconsistent. It seems to me to be the ethical equivalent of using patients as means to fulfill the formal requirements of principles rather than using principles as means towards understanding just what respecting a patient as an end in himself amounts to in any particular case. Is it possible that we have become so focused on trying to satisfy the narrow, formal requirements of the principles of autonomy, non-maleficence and beneficence in such problematic situations that we fail to see the "system errors"—i.e., the social arrangements that directly contribute to the kinds of inequities and insensitivities that so threaten the quality of the lives of patients?

Once again, insofar as the health care team regards the social aspects of the case, especially the social disposition of elderly patients who need mild to moderate physical assistance, they encounter these aspects as ready-made and unchallengeable givens. Most communities are unable, unwilling or do not have reason to believe that they are ethically obligated to commit social resources towards developing feasible strategies to encourage patients such as this man to feel included as a positively valued part of the community. In such an environment, there is no compelling reason for this man to believe that he ought to stay alive. Thus, the "problem" for the clinicians and this patient is, to a significant degree, pre-set by the community's patterns of actions and beliefs, over which the principle agents in this case perceive themselves to have little, if any, control. The situation is thus perceived as a conflict between the principle of autonomy (i.e., the patient's) and the principles of beneficence and non-maleficence (i.e., the clinicians' pursuit of what they consider to be their professional goals).

In the analysis of this case in chapter two, it was noted that it may very well be possible for the clinicians to elicit from the patient a coherent account of his behavior and that this should be attempted. But more is needed. The patient should not only be challenged to give reasons for his behavior; but the clinicians ought also to call into question the tacit attitudes and behavior of the community's treatment of its indigent and physically impaired elderly. That is, the reconstructed approach proposed here would require the health care team to examine critically the social "givens," such as communities' obligations to their older members.

Take, for example, the socio-cultural issue of sustenance. This man chose to quit eating and drinking—very possibly the only means available to him to carry out his intentions—and eating and drinking are emotionally charged activities for clinicians and laypersons alike. Though often difficult to read off of the surface features of current cultural practices, eating and drinking are still considered highly symbolic activities—despite the significant evolution that the eating and drinking habits of the younger generations in the United States today have undergone. The act of eating and drinking together symbolizes intimacy, trust, acceptance among strangers. All cultures are permeated with examples of the symbolism of eating and drinking. A toast, breaking bread together, communion—all represent the primordial need to recognize the existence of self in other and other in self. All of these symbolize our essential interconnectedness. Transpose this symbolism to this man's case...what is his refusal to eat and drink saying to his caregivers? to his community? to his culture? to us? And what does allowing him to refuse until he becomes semi-conscious say—both to him and to the rest of us—about the meaning of our response?

Clinicians provide an invaluable service to the rest of the community when, through their unique experiences, they are able to bear witness—not silently, but vocally—to the burdensomeness of the consequences of certain social arrangements that might otherwise go unnoticed or unheeded until much later, if at all. In a responsive and responsible democracy, such "problematic situations" are best resolved by being brought to the public's attention, where they can be addressed and reconstructed from a truly broad and representative bio/psycho/social perspective—and at the earliest opportunity. For example, the alternative approach could lead us to consider, on the basis of its particular bio/psycho/social interpretation of individualism, that the decisional capacity of this man has, in fact, been impaired. The reasoning might proceed as follows. Based on the five criteria described on page 26 of chapter two—i.e., understanding, rationality, opportunity, absence from coercion and authenticity—this man has not been adequately protected from an external form of coercion, namely, the alienating and inhospitable environmental (i.e., social) conditions. (The fact that these conditions are the result of our society's current prejudicial disregard of the elderly is an additional, but separate concern.) Because of this, the authenticity of his decision and present pattern of behavior—a key element of autonomy—might be challenged. However, in questioning this man's decisional capacity in this manner, clinicians will open up therewith the possibility of questioning the social conditions responsible for creating the external coercion leading to this man's psychological disposition. That is, once the broader perspective is taken, the clinicians cannot then return to the standard approach and its focus on individual decision-making at that point.

But, again, what this broader approach rests on is the development of a different set of presuppositions about persons and a different way of framing norms, practices, commitments, expectations and reciprocity between individuals and the social institutions they create. And, doing so, again, requires replacing a reactionary applications model of medical and ethical problem-solving with one that is participatory, prospective and able to move beyond a crisis mode to one of prevention. A first step in the transformation of the way in which health care institutions currently function might be to create a variety of interdisciplinary deliberative and advisory bodies. These bodies or councils would function as a communicative bridge between the various social institutions, professional experts and the public. They would make possible a continuous, prospective monitoring and critique of the strengths and weaknesses of the available services of existing social institutions and of the presence or absence of a healthy variety of strategies for their access by all of the community's members.

Just how this step might transform the options of a patient like the one in the present case is only hypothetical because, as yet, these are not live alternatives that can actually be offered in this particular case. Until these prospective modifications are actually available and tried—in the *doing* and its consequences as opposed to the necessary, but still merely preliminary speculative brainstorming—so that the extent of their effects can be measured, assessed and compared to what we would hope to achieve, their efficacy will remain an open question. However, the alternative approach suggested here makes it possible to offer a more realistic account of the bio/psycho/social realities of this case and requires us to keep searching for practical ways to respect such bio/psycho/social realities in the actions we take. This approach, by keeping the antecedents and consequents of issues open to potential inquiry, prevents the resolutions of specific cases from becoming reified and regarded as a variety of standard practice that is so fixed that it is impervious to future, critical examination and revision. Parenthetically, it also prevents or, at least, attenuates the tendency to regard the social *status quo* as an unfortunate circumstance beyond control—a falsely comforting, but particularly vicious sentimentality we cannot long afford, as individuals, as professionals or as a society.

2.3 Case 3: Hyperacute Rejection Syndrome

A 26 year old woman developed myocarditis (a severely damaging inflammation of the heart which interferes with the ability of the heart to pump blood efficiently) during an otherwise unremarkable pregnancy. Although she eventually delivered a premature but viable and healthy infant, the patient's own cardiac function deteriorated to the point where a transplant was the only remaining chance for saving her life. After delivery, a properly matched donor heart eventually became available and she underwent a transplantation that involved no immediate complications.

Several hours post-transplant and while still in the recovery room, the patient's cardiac function rapidly began to deteriorate. It was apparent that she was experiencing a "hyperacute rejection" (a process of organ transplant rejection whose etiology is poorly understood and which in about 95% of cases leads to repeat rejection should another transplant be attempted). The patient was placed on mechanical pump support as the newly transplanted heart could no longer provide the pumping action required to keep the patient alive. While she is currently awake, able to speak and rational, the mechanical pump is, at its present stage of technological development, only a stop-gap measure. Therefore, if this patient does not receive another heart transplant, she will die.

When a heart that is a good match for this patient finally becomes available, it also happens to be an equally good match for another potential recipient who is awaiting transplant for the first time. The hospital ethics committee is asked whether the transplant team should re-transplant this patient or give the heart to the other waiting candidate.

2.3.1 Analysis

The analysis of this case in chapter two ended with the transplant team in the unenviable position of having to choose between a number of conflicting ethical obligations: (1) to the patient with hyperacute rejection syndrome, (2) to the other potential first-time recipient (who has a significantly greater chance of survival), (3) to their profession and (4) to the community. After weighing the implications of what the principles of autonomy, beneficence, non-maleficence and justice seemed to require, the team decided that, all things considered, offering re-transplantation to the patient with hyperacute rejection syndrome was the most compelling of their obligations. The rationale behind the decision was based on a utilitarian argument to the effect that their decision would, overall, preserve the greatest number of interests and values that these conflicting principles are said to under-write.

However, once again, the health care professionals involved in this case are presented with a set of conflicting social expectations arising from social structures the majority of which they have no available mechanisms for challenging. In today's understanding of the transplant team/patient relationship and through the institutions that embody that understanding, the team is virtually compelled to re-transplant the patient with hyperacute rejection. On the other hand, it is increasingly the community's tacit assumption that the proper role of health care professionals includes gatekeeping at the bedside, in which clinicians are expected to be responsible for efficient resource allocation at the bedside on a case-by-case basis. Clearly there is a clash of principles at work here and present thinking includes no "super-principle," no fixed precedence principle that can be applied in the event that principles conflict.

Obviously, in any scenario where scarce resources require the adoption of some kind of distribution scheme, gate-keeping must occur. However, for a distribution scheme to have any degree of accuracy, effectiveness and equity, it is necessary for the person or group of persons responsible for the distribution to have the same general, impersonal relationship with and obligations to *all* of the potential beneficiaries. While there is no doubt that the information generated at the bedside is necessary for the kind of data accumulation required in order to provide an equitable global system of distribution, it is quite illogical to conclude that the appropriate distribution of scarce resources therefore, can occur at the bedside. Thus, while clinicians, by virtue of their special expertise, have an obligation to serve as technical advisors to the community, they simply cannot, by virtue of their special relationships with identified patients, be expected to act simultaneously as fair and impersonal gate-keepers. Only someone or some group having access to all of the relevant information available and capable of adequately and fairly representing *all* the potential beneficiaries should be performing this role.

It is the case that, whenever a person applies a principle, follows a rule, assumes a role, etc., she is tacitly endorsing the commitments implied by those activities. That is, a clinician's willing—even if grudging—participation in gate-keeping at the bedside implies that she accepts this practice as one of her legitimate roles and, accordingly, will assume responsibility for the consequences of her actions. The fact that she recognizes there is a conflict of interests and principles occurring signals the beginning of critical, reflective thought. Pitting each interest and principle against one another and weighing the consequences without attempting to subject the implications of the particular antecedents and consequents of the case to careful scrutiny circumvents controlled inquiry and replaces it with the ethical equivalent of following the path of least resistance. To maintain, upon critical reflection, that following such a path is not, in fact, a choice is to engage (at best) in naive self-deception or worse, in cynical pretense. Acquiescence—just like "choosing not to choose"—is, in fact, a choice—and it can be quite an ethically significant one at that.

Accordingly, as has been argued in the previous two cases, ethical obligation is not a one-way street. In the tacit relationship that exists between clinicians and communities, if a change on one side of the relationship occurs, and is not questioned or rejected by the others parties involved, it is not unreasonable to presume that it is an accepted—or at least tolerated—change. That is why it is so crucial that clinicians have recourse to some mechanism by which they can challenge the ethical appropriateness of society's demands upon them respecting issues such as this one. A bio/psycho/social approach opens the possibility of questioning the "givens" of such issues by making explicit the implicit—and often surprisingly contradictory—presuppositions behind social aspects of cases, aspects that have been tacitly accepted, if not explicitly endorsed, as social practices. Rather than being presented with a *fait accompli* that ends inquiry and requires a futile and fruitless engagement in post hoc justification, clinicians can concentrate on much more positive and productive efforts. These efforts would include helping to create more equitable arrangements for the distribution of medical benefits and burdens and of other social goods and services.

In the immediacy of any particular patient's crisis, of course, there is no time to put a broad socially responsible decision-making process in place to determine the proper use of scarce transplant resources. But that only means that clinicians who strive to do their ethical reflection using a bio/psycho/social approach rather than continuing to rely on the standard approach, must begin well in advance of such crises. In fact they must begin now. They must critique and seek modification of institutional structures and practices that foreclose the full actualization of the possibilities this alternative approach reveals. And, personal commitment, while absolutely essential, is simply not enough here. Confronting system errors—which is precisely what these sorts of issues are—requires collective effort. This is where this country's ingrained patterns of "rugged individualism" can actually become quite counterproductive—we simply don't have a track-record of trusting one another long enough to appreciate what collective action can accomplish. Libertarian assumptions notwithstanding, being co-opted is not an inevitable consequence of engaging in collective action!

3. THE ETHICS COMMITTEE: RESOLUTION OR FURTHER SYMPTOM?

One response to the present ethical difficulties facing patient/clinician relationships is the ethics committee. Historically such committees have been constituted by individual health care facilities to help their staff, their patients and a very circumscribed local community to make better informed decisions about the specific health care options offered by that facility. And, certainly, there is evidence to suggest that ethics committees, when properly organized and prepared, are eminently suited to the task. They can provide the sort of forum in which disparately functioning social institutions can be co-ordinated to benefit maximally both health care as a social institution as well as the public it serves.[5]

However, the majority of ethics committees currently functioning in this country are hamstrung by the same sorts of difficulties already described as burdening and limiting health care delivery. They are hamstrung by isolation, by insulation, by being co-opted by special interests and, most importantly, by being confronted with piece-meal, ready-made, socially-induced (or exacerbated) problems that individually need resolution on an emergency basis. That is, they face the same sort of *faits accomplis* that are so detrimental to the effectiveness of social institutions in general and health care professionals in particular.

This difficulty is made most evident when we compare an idealization of the most effective ethics committee with the way in which most ethics committees currently function. Ideally speaking an ethics committee has three functions: education, policy consultation and case consultation (listed in order of importance). More specifically, these functions can be described as including:

1. *Education*: in the course of educating itself, it also educates health care staff, patient/clients, their significant others and the community at large about ethical issues in general as well as those specifically affecting the relationships between the facility and its community of staff and patients/clients
2. *Policy consultation*: it assists with institutional policy review by helping to develop, review and up-date the facility's health care policies in light of the community's needs
3. *Case consultation*: it provides expertise and support for health care staff, patient/clients and their significant others in health care decision-making by helping all of the parties concerned to develop the insight necessary to identify and analyse aspects of individual cases that have become ethically troubling and to suggest strategies for their resolution that would not be ethically inappropriate

Though our experience with ethics committees in this country is, as yet, somewhat limited, it still suggests that, when these responsibilities are conscientiously met, in this particular order of importance, a committee's ability to devise preventive strategies actually succeeds within the institution. Moreover, it minimizes the need to devise reactionary or defensive strategies for the constant, superficial and purely symptomatic treatment of full-blown ethical conflicts and dilemmas. That is, when the first two functions are adequately met, the third function requires a relatively little investment of time and effort. When the last responsibility is the only one emphasized—which is far too often the case with many existing ethics committees—it becomes impossible for a committee to control inquiry sufficiently to provide anything more substantial than an unsatisfying "quick fix." That is, it can provide only a temporary, piece-meal and already polarized standard approach-based solution to problems already "given." Ethics committees that choose to deal only with the last function in this reactionary manner are left in precisely the same situation as the little Dutch boy with his finger in the dike. They will never get beyond that last function to deal with the first two functions. And these are the only preventive strategies that have a chance of effectively dealing with ethical issues prospectively and resolving specific, concrete cases via controlled, systematic and progressive inquiry.

Every effort must be made to avoid this situation for several extremely important reasons. The first is a technical consideration: as I have argued, the problem as "given" is outside of controlled inquiry insofar as it offers no guarantee of an adequate assessment of the roots of an issue. That is, even though ethics committees *can* play an important role in responsible decision-making as described in the previous section, they are often not able to do so. Too often existing forces within their institution divert them away from the first two roles and into an exclusive—or nearly so—preoccupation with the third. The second reason is really the more central, as it involves an ethical consideration: when an ethics committee allows itself to become preoccupied with case consultations to the point that it virtually ignores all else, something strange threatens. The committee is tempted to see itself less as a consultative body that attempts to provide logical and conceptual clarity and support to the deliberations between clinicians and patients, and more as the deliberative body itself. Look to the not-so-subtle changes reflected in the language: instead of marshalling a range of alternatives that are "not ethically inappropriate," ethical principles are hauled out to "justify the best course of action to be taken." This begins to sound more like a pronouncement (from on high?), than an attempt to provide conceptual clarity or practical guidelines to those relevantly affected in their search for a range of ethically sensitive possibilities.

Another related feature of ethics committees that can actively create difficulties is composition. Most always the composition of an ethics committee consists largely of persons who are employed by or have, whether directly or indirectly, some financial relationship with the medical facility within which the committee exists. For this reason it is extremely important that the members of such committees are sufficiently shielded from any real or perceived pressure from the parent facility, and can meticulously avoid the inevitable, sometimes quite subtle and oftentimes innocent bias or misplaced loyalty they may feel for their workplace community. There need be no inherent conflict of interest, so long as those relevantly affected by the influence of the committee are sufficiently represented. To that end, my ethicist colleague, Erich H. Loewy, and I have always strongly urged those facilities for whom we have provided ethics education and consultation to seek out as broad a representation from the local community as possible. Such a committee should include representation not only from pastoral care, nursing, allied health care, social services and the various clinical departments of the facility, but from community members *outside* of the facility as well: laypersons from various walks of life, lawyers, other clergy representatives, minority groups, non-medical academics, etc. For example, when there is to be only one legal representative on such a committee, it is crucial that she *not* be one of the facility's lawyers. This may seem like a "no-brainer," but it is amazing how many lawyers on hospital ethics committees have some kind of pecuniary relationship with the hospital! Clearly, this could create a real or perceived ethical conflict of interest and, so, should be studiously avoided.

One of the more disturbing trends of late has been the introduction of an "ethics presence" into some of the private or "semi-private" corporations and health maintenance-related organizations in this country (I include under "semi"-private any organization that receives *any* public funding). This has occurred in both for-profit and not-for-profit institutions, and involves either the hiring of "corporate" ethicists or the creation of ethics committees—or both—with the specific aim of defending and/or promulgating the particular philosophy of the parent institution or organization. In and of itself, this is not ethically problematic, so long as the agenda of these corporate entities is public knowledge and they are introduced to complement, rather than replace, the open and democratically representative ethics committee described above. However, when the deliberations of an ethics advisor or ethics committee must comply with—or is any way constrained by—a narrower philosophy than that held by the individuals it is established to counsel, it is no longer appropriate to consider either these entities or their deliberations as involving "ethics," and to treat them as such is, in itself, ethically suspect. Call these entities what they, in fact, are—morals counselors or morals committees—and *not* ethics counselors or ethics committees.

The development of ethics committees—and the continual improvement of existing ones through patient, facility, community and committee education—can be one hopeful move towards the reconstruction of social institutions and facilities that are more sensitive to the needs of the individuals they serve. But, again, *unless and until presuppositions about persons and their relationships are also routinely subjected to critical reflection, our attempts at reconstructing the social structures themselves will lack the precision they might otherwise have.* Until this fact is fully appreciated, most of our ethical thinking in health care ethics will remain unaffected—and far less effective that it could be.

4. INCORPORATING A BIO/PSYCHO/SOCIAL APPROACH AND PERSPECTIVE INTO DAILY CLINICAL PRACTICE

One of the frequent issues I've encountered in discussions with clinicians is their concern that the alternative approach I offer does not provide enough explicit direction to help them incorporate it into their daily practice. Were this the whole of their concern—and further discussion often reveals it is not—it is easily enough remedied in the course of reviewing with them a sample "work-up guide," the most recent of which I shall include and discuss in more detail at the end of this section. Used as an example of what an apt ethical decision-making model ought to include, it represents, in briefest outline, a number of years' experience discussing methodological considerations in ethical decision-making with health care clinicians from a wide variety of backgrounds.

However, the problem for these clinicians is usually a deeper, far more ingrained concern, viz., to be able to see a rather dramatic improvement over the traditional approach, a measurable improvement from which they—and their patients—can immediately benefit. This concern, of course, is not as easily remedied. Even if the entire society suddenly adopted a bio/psycho/social approach and became critically and prospectively reflective (unfortunately, a rather unrealistic scenario), *overt* measurable benefits would not be immediate. This would prove to be the case especially in those cases where it is the social—i.e., institutional—aspects of the case that are problematic and in need of reconstruction. We are, unfortunately, a society which has perpetrated—and then whole-heartedly bought into—the myth of "the clean, quick fix," as though a circumscribed solution is simply standing by, ready to the hand of each individual who possesses but the insight and industry to "apply" it. Our current government's penchant for "surgical strikes" by the military is one that comes most immediately to mind here.

The gravest problem with such thinking is the behavior and attitudes it spawns: the "application" solves the "problem" and leaves no "residue;" agent, means and ends or goals are rendered clear and distinct, external to, independent of and, thus, unaffected by each other. Of course, I am not saying that surgical strikes are to no effect. But, just as our military experience ought to have taught us, there *is* a "residue," and it can have profound untoward effects—some more telling than others. In other words, agents, means and ends or goals are much like integrated circuitry. That is, they are integrally interconnected: whenever agents make choices (and remember, *not* choosing *is* a choice), they, too, are changed in the process. The change may not, at first, be overt; but change occurs, nonetheless. And, experience teaches us that the changes of which we are unaware are always those we least control.

Resolving problems in such a way as to better understand and control the antecedent conditions that gave rise to the situation in the first place as well as the consequences of both the problem and our attempts to remedy it simply requires more time. It does so if only because it both necessitates and is necessary for a readjustment of both personal and social habits. Not only do these readjustments take time, so does a reassessment of the long-term effects of the readjustments themselves. What this approach can promise when carried out systematically and consistently is slow, but progressive improvement in the quality of our communal existence. Such an improvement is the necessary though, perhaps, not sufficient condition for the possibility of improving *all*, and not just some, of our individual, personal lives—the means to which the traditional approach, for all it's emphasis on individualism, respect and human dignity, still largely misses.

5. A SAMPLE HEALTH CARE ETHICS WORKUP GUIDE

This health care ethics workup guide remains a work in progress. It is offered as but one example of how one might distill from the discipline of ethics a systematic approach—as opposed to a fixed tablet of ready-made principles or laws—to inquiry into ethically problematic cases and issues:

1. Begin to describe—by representing as many relevant perspectives as possible—all of the facts of the case or issue: environmental, biological, psychological and social
2. Ascertain who is being treated and, if not the patient, assess the legitimacy of such treatment

3. Determine the legitimate decision-maker(s)—not always an easy thing to ascertain, and not always the same as the person(s) being treated—and stand ready to give compelling reasons for this choice
4. Describe the relevant values and interests of the health care team, the patient, the significant others and/or family, the relevant social institutions and the society itself
5. Examine the ways in which these various important values and interests are interrelated
6. Determine various possible courses of action that are not ethically inappropriate and that are protective of as many values and interests in the case as possible
7. Discuss the alternative choices and their implications, including what would count as benefits and drawbacks from the perspectives of those most relevantly affected
8. Stand ready to give a well-reasoned defense of the course or courses of action you think most appropriate for resolving the issue
9. Be willing to question and re-assess, at any time, any aspects of the particular case or issue in question, including the decision-making process itself

6. CONCLUDING REMARKS

My aim in this work has been to examine critically a standard approach to the process of identifying, analysing and resolving problematic cases in the field of health care ethics. In the course this examination, certain presuppositions that are central to this approach have been identified, and their antecedents and consequents (i.e., origin, function and implications) explored. These presuppositions concern the nature of persons, describing as "given," or essential, attributes that are, in reality, the result of a particular strain of human development. The results of this examination suggest that this set of unreflectively held presuppositions is indicative of a deeper, uncritically held methodological presupposition: namely, that there are aspects of experience that can be fixed and captured by language, conceptualized into principles and then "applied" in algorithmic fashion to solve problems.

In this work I have offered an alternative approach to patient/clinician encounters which, while it does not abandon principles, argues that principles, applied without understanding the bio/psycho/social dynamics of a particular case can cause us to miss much that is central to that encounter. The alternative approach advocated in this work rejects the notion that problematic issues or cases can be settled "even-handedly" by largely ignoring the specific bio/psycho/social features and contextual differences of situations and applying the same generic principles and considerations equally to all persons.. Instead, it seeks resolution to ethically problematic cases by attempting to understand the complex interrelationships that have developed between patients and their entire intellectual, emotional, social and material environment, including significant others, caregivers, communities and cultures. It seeks to devise prospective, as opposed to reactionary, strategies capable of resolving, as early as possible, conflicts that will inevitably arise in the course of these interrelationships. In so doing, this approach denies the validity of ethical behavior based on the "application" of either static principles or individualistic and subjective intuitions.

My account denies the possibility of understanding either the individual or community in isolation from one another. They are not rigid or static and isolated conceptions, but fluid and dynamic interrelationships *within* the organism/environment complex. The integrity of each of the parts is, therefore, dependent upon activities that promote the continued integrity and solidarity of the whole. This requires the co-operation of persons in recognizing, communicating, and respecting each others' bio/psycho/social realities and perspectives as providing a uniquely necessary element so essential to the intelligent (which includes ethical) direction and integration of our personal habits as well as our social practices, customs and institutions.

ENDNOTES

1. Edmund D. Pellegrino and David C. Thomasma, *For the Patient's Good: The Restoration of Beneficence in Health Care* (New York: Oxford University Press), 1988.
2. One of the most prominent physicians of the nineteenth century was Rudolf Virchow, the father of pathology, who campaigned vigorously for social reforms and, on more than one occasion, annoyed the government of Germany by criticizing the existing social conditions. In the 1920's, Margaret Higgins Sanger, a nurse and founder of the birth control movement in the United States, was harassed, jailed and generally vilified by the government
3. Nurses Alliance for the Prevention of Nuclear War, Physicians for Social Responsibility and International Physicians for the Prevention of Nuclear War are three organizations that come immediately to mind.
4. This lack might help to explain—though hardly justify—why, for example, health care providers passively tolerated for nearly twenty years reports published in some of the most prestigious medical journals by the United States Public Health Services concerning their Tuskegee "study," which consisted of placing over two hundred syphilitic black men on placebos, allowing them to believe they were being given state-of-the-art treatment, and purposely trying to thwart their receiving effective treatment from any other source. It was 1973 before the United States Public Health Services called an end to this technically- as well as ethically- flawed study. There are now a number of excellent sources for the history of this, and other, unconscionable practices that have, at one time or another, been tolerated under the rubric of medical experimentation. For Tuskegee, see especially the classic history by James H. Jones, *Bad Blood: The Tuskegee Syphilis*

Experiment (New York: Free Press), 1981 and the section featured in *The Hastings Center Report,* vol. 22, no. 6, Nov-Dec, 1992, pp. 29-40.

5. A relatively unique example of the creation of such a forum devoted to sustained prospective inquiry into a specific, but wide-ranging ethical issue in health care is the President's Commission for the Study of Ethical Problems in Medicine and Biomedical and Behavioral Research. Their publication, *Deciding to Forego Life-Sustaining Treatment: A Report of the Ethical, Medical and Legal Issues in Treatment Decisions*, March, 1983, illustrates the potential fruits of the creation of such fora. However, one of the main drawbacks of this commission was a failure to establish or at least encourage mechanisms of public dialogue to respond to the commission, which consisted almost entirely of Ph.D.'s, JDs MD's and one or two Jesuits. The results of such a commission should mark the beginning of public education, dialogue, synthesis and the eventual launching of carefully monitored and studied experimental programs, and not merely the end of philosophical analysis

Select Bibliography

JOHN DEWEY

Boydston, Jo Ann, ed. *John Dewey: The Early Works, 1882-1898*. Vol. 5 (1895-1898): "The Reflex Arc Concept in Psychology." *Early Essays*. Carbondale: Southern Illinois University Press, 1972: 96-109.

Boydston, Jo Ann, ed. *John Dewey: The Middle Works, 1899-1924*. Vol. 3 (1903): "Logical Conditions of a Scientific Treatment of Morality." *Essays of the New Empiricism*. Carbondale: Southern Illinois University Press, 1977: 3-39.

Boydston, Jo Ann, ed. *John Dewey: The Middle Works, 1899-1924*. Vol. 12 (1920): *Reconstruction in Philosophy and Essays*. Carbondale: Southern Illinois University Press, 1988: 77-201.

Boydston, Jo Ann, ed. *John Dewey: The Middle Works, 1899-1924*. Vol. 14 (1922): *Human Nature and Conduct*. Carbondale: Southern Illinois University Press, 1988.

Boydston, Jo Ann, ed. *John Dewey: The Later Works, 1925-1953*. Vol. 1 (1925): *Experience and Nature*. Chaps. 5, 6 and 7. Carbondale: Southern Illinois University Press, 1988.

Boydston, Jo Ann, ed. *John Dewey: The Later Works, 1925-1953*. Vol. 2 (1925-1927): *The Public and Its Problems*. Carbondale: Southern Illinois University Press, 1988: 235-372.

Boydston, Jo Ann, ed. *John Dewey: The Later Works, 1925-1953*. Vol. 4 (1929): *The Quest for Certainty*. Carbondale: Southern Illinois University Press, 1988.

Boydston, Jo Ann, ed. *John Dewey: The Later Works, 1925-1953*. Vol. 5 (1929-1930): *Individualism, Old and New*. Carbondale: Southern Illinois University Press, 1988: 41-123.

Boydston, Jo Ann, ed. *John Dewey: The Later Works, 1925-1953*. Vol. 10 (1934): *Art as Experience*. Chap. 3. Carbondale: Southern Illinois University Press, 1989.

Boydston, Jo Ann, ed. *John Dewey: The Later Works, 1925-1953*. Vol. 12 (1938): *Logic: The Theory of Inquiry*. Carbondale: Southern Illinois University Press, 1991.

Gouinlock, James. *Excellence in Public Discourse: John Stuart Mill, John Dewey and Social Intelligence*. New York: Teachers College Press, 1986.

Rucker, Darnell. "Selves into Persons: Another Legacy from John Dewey." *Rice University Studies*. Vol. 66, no. 4 (Fall, 1980): pp. 103-118.

Stuhr, John J. *Classical American Philosophy: Essential Readings and Interpretive Essays.* New York: Oxford University Press, 1987.
Westbrook, Robert B. *John Dewey and American Democracy.* London: Cornell University Press, 1991.

FEMINIST LITERATURE

Canadian Feminist Ethics Theory Group: Lorraine Code, Maureen Ford, Kathleen Martindale, Susan Sherwin and Debra Shogan. "Some Issues in the Ethics of Collaborative Work." *Explorations in Feminist Ethics.* Ed. Eve Browning Cole and Susan Coultrap-McQuin. Bloomington: Indiana University Press, 1992: 131-7.
Code, Lorraine. "Persons and Others." *Power, Gender, Values.* Ed. Judith Genova. Edmonton: Academic Printing and Publishing, 1987:143-71.
Cole, Eve Browning. *Philosophy and Feminist Criticism: An Introduction.* New York: Paragon House, 1993.
Dillon, Robin S. "Care and Respect." *Explorations in Feminist Ethics.* Ed. Eve Browning Cole and Susan Coultrap-McQuin. Bloomington: Indiana University Press, 1992: 69-81.
Dillon, Robin S. "Respect and Care: Toward Moral Integration." *Canadian Journal of Philosophy.* Vol. 22, no. 1 (March, 1992): 105-32.
Seigfried, Charlene H. "Pragmatism, Feminism and Sensitivity to Context." *Who Cares? Theory, Research and Educational Implications of the Ethic of Care.* Ed. Mary M. Brabeck. New York: Praeger, 1989: 63-83.
Walker, Margaret Urban. "Moral Understandings: Alternative 'Epistemology' for a Feminist Ethics." *Explorations in Feminist Ethics.* Ed. Eve Browning Cole and Susan Coultrap-McQuin.Bloomington: Indiana University Press, 1992: 165-75.
Whitbeck, Caroline. "A Different Reality: Feminist Ontology." *Beyond Domination: New Perspectives on Women and Philosophy.* Ed. Carol Gould. Totowa, N.J.: Rowman and Allenheld, 1983: 64-85.

OTHER PERTINENT LITERATURE IN MEDICINE AND PHILOSOPHY:

Engelhardt, H.T. *Foundations of Bioethics.* New York: Oxford University Press, 1986: 68-135.
Habermas, Jurgen. *Moral Consciousness and Communicative Action.* Cambridge, Massachusetts: MIT Press, 1990: 116-194.
Loewy, Erich H. *Suffering and the Beneficent Community.* New York: State University of New York Press, 1991.
Loewy, Erich H. *Freedom and Community.* New York: State University of New York Press, 1993.
Moreno, Jonathan D. "The Social Individual in Clinical Ethics." *Journal of Clinical Ethics,* vol. 3, N. 1 (1992): 53-5.
Ozar, David T. and Sokol, David J. *Dental Ethics At Chairside: Professional Principles and Practical Applications* New York: Mosby-Yearbook, Inc., 1994.
Pellegrino, Edmund D. and Thomasma, David C. *For the Patient's Good: The Restoration of Beneficence in Health Care* New York: Oxford University Press, 1988.

Reich, Warren T., ed. *Encyclopedia of Bioethics: Revised Edition*. New York: Simon & Schuster Macmillan, 1995.
Rosenthal, Sandra B. "Foundations, Rationality and Intelligent Responsibility: A Pragmatic Perspective." *Reason Papers*. 16(Fall, 1991): 73-94.
Szasz, Thomas S. and Hollender, Marc H. "A Contribution to the Philosophy of Medicine: The Basic Models of the Doctor-Patient Relationship." *Archives of Internal Medicine*. Vol. 97 (1956): 585-92.
Thomasma, David C. and Graber, Glenn C. *Theory and Practice in Medical Ethics*. New York: Continuum, 1989.
Veach, Robert M. "Models for Ethical Medicine in a Revolutionary Age." *Hastings Center Report*, June, 1972: 5-7.

Index

MIX
Papier aus verantwortungsvollen Quellen
Paper from responsible sources
FSC® C105338

FSC
www.fsc.org

If you have any concerns about our products,
you can contact us on
ProductSafety@springernature.com

In case Publisher is established outside the EU,
the EU authorized representative is:
Springer Nature Customer Service Center GmbH
Europaplatz 3, 69115 Heidelberg, Germany

Printed by Libri Plureos GmbH
in Hamburg, Germany